An Introduction to Embodied Mind is a terrific introductory text on the philosophy of embodied and extended cognition. The authors bring philosophical issues to life through intriguing real-world examples and case studies, explicitly addressing applied topics of ethical and personal significance alongside their coherent and powerful framework in philosophy of mind. A focused line of thought is established over the course of the book, even while the authors give fair attention to approaches which diverge from their preferred one. Students in all areas of Philosophy, as well as other researchers interested in embodied cognition, will enjoy and benefit from this book.

John Sutton, *Professor in Philosophy at Stirling University, Scotland*

AN INTRODUCTION TO EMBODIED MIND

An Introduction to Embodied Mind: Thinking Outside the Head offers readers a valuable gateway to understanding one of the most exciting ideas in philosophy and cognitive science: that minds are not confined to the brain but extend into the body and environment. Written in a clear, engaging style, the book guides readers through competing views of embodiment and shows how they matter for everyday life.

The book is divided into three parts. Part 1 begins with familiar ideas about mind–body separation and gradually leads readers toward embodied perspectives, distinguishing between "weak" and "strong" versions of embodiment. Part 2 develops two influential approaches to embodied cognition and highlights their strengths as well as their challenges. Part 3 explores how these theories make a difference in practice, with applications to free will, ethics, technology, and cultural life.

Each chapter includes accessible overviews, exercises in "Otto's Workbook" that encourage active reflection, and "Sidequests" and "The More You Know" boxes that invite readers to dig deeper. Examples are drawn from popular culture, psychology, and everyday experience, making the material approachable for students and general readers alike.

With its blend of rigorous philosophy, practical exercises, and lively examples—as well as a helpful glossary—*An Introduction to Embodied Mind: Thinking Outside the Head* provides an engaging exploration of embodiment for anyone curious about how minds really work.

Aaron Kagan is a user experience researcher and strategist with over a decade of experience designing and studying complex human–technology systems. He has held staff-level research roles at Google, Meta, and other technology companies, including work across Search, extended reality, and emerging AI systems. He is the founder of GraspingAI, a consultancy focused on human-centered AI, and has served in leadership roles within the American Philosophical Association supporting non-academic and industry careers.

Charles Lassiter is Professor of Philosophy at Gonzaga University. His areas of research include philosophy of mind and social epistemology, focusing on issues at the intersection of cognition and culture. He also collects and analyzes data about the academic philosophy job market.

AN INTRODUCTION TO EMBODIED MIND

Thinking Outside the Head

Aaron Kagan and Charles Lassiter

Routledge
Taylor & Francis Group
NEW YORK AND LONDON

Designed cover image: Sam Kagan Art

First published 2026
by Routledge
605 Third Avenue, New York, NY 10158

and by Routledge
4 Park Square, Milton Park, Abingdon, Oxon, OX14 4RN

Routledge is an imprint of the Taylor & Francis Group, an informa business

ISBN: 978-1-032-41178-1 (hbk)
ISBN: 978-1-032-41177-4 (pbk)
ISBN: 978-1-003-35662-2 (ebk)

DOI: 10.4324/9781003356622

Typeset in Sabon
by SPi Technologies India Pvt Ltd (Straive)

CONTENTS

To the reader ix
Gratitude xiii

PART 1
Framing the question **1**

1 Introduction 3

2 From aporia to philosophy 7

3 The rise and fall of disembodiment 18

4 The extended mind 47

PART 2
Refining the theories **65**

5 Interlude 67

6 Interpretations of the extended mind 72

7 Weak embodied cognition 85

8 Objections to weak embodied cognition 101

9 Strong embodiment 111

10 Objections to strong embodiment 142

PART 3
Applications and extensions **149**

11 Interlude: Exposition to application 151

12 Free will, determinism, and embodiment 156

13 Ethics and embodiment 180

14 Technology and embodiment 199

15 Future directions 212

Works cited *220*
Suggested reading *225*
Glossary *230*
Index *250*

TO THE READER

We wrote this book to introduce the embodied mind in a way that's accessible to everyone, especially university students. It can be enjoyed "as is" or paired as part of a university course.

Here are a few things we've done to help with these use cases.

Structure of the book

In this book, we're going to think through how the body and mind are related to one another and how that makes us what we are. We focus on one particular answer to that question: minds are **embodied**. Another way of putting this is to say that thinking doesn't just happen "in our heads" but that the mind *extends* out into the world.[1] What does that mean? It means that bodies are a crucial part of the story for how the mind works. How we think, feel, and experience the world—the body plays a key role in all of it, and more.

Who is this book for? Anyone with a mind and body and a little curiosity about what makes us the kinds of thinking things we are.[2]

How does the book work? It's broken up into three parts. In Part 1, we show how we move from "mind over matter" and "matter over mind" to ideas about embodiment. There are a lot of different ways to think about embodiment, and we're going to try to help make sense of them. We'll separate ideas about embodiment into two camps: strong and weak. In Part 2, we'll develop two varieties of embodied cognition (and express some worries about them). In Part 3, we'll see how these different ideas about embodiment make a difference in the world, especially for topics like free will, ethics, and technology.

Every chapter begins with a Chapter Overview. It provides a brief guide to the ideas and topics you can expect to encounter. Throughout the book, you'll find terms that are in boldface type. These include useful bits of jargon and also names of philosophers and psychologists who have made big contributions to our understanding of embodiment.

Speaking of chapters, you'll find a few different kinds of set-out boxes. There's **Otto's workbook**. These are exercises to do to help explore some of the ideas. (In Chapter 4, you'll see why we use the name "Otto.") Then we have **Sidequests**: we give you some pointers to related topics and ask you to do some poking around. These are typically a bit more advanced. Finally, we have **The More You Know**. These go deeper into some particular topics that are brought up in the reading. You can get by with reading the main text and skipping these boxes, but we hope you'll take the time to do some of them. Philosophy is active, not passive. Your experience of reading this book will be richer if you engage with it.

The flow of the book is intended to take readers from intuitive and conflicting ideas about the mind to varieties of embodiment. If you're a philosopher of mind (or have had to suffer through a conversation with one), you might raise an eyebrow that we're beginning with disembodiment. This is an intentional choice. It seems like disembodiment is the default position for many people when it comes to thinking about the nature of the mind. From *Freaky Friday*'s body swapping to uploading your consciousness to a computer—these examples assume that the mind is disembodied in some way. There's some research to suggest that this is fairly widespread across cultures.[3] Maybe we're born thinking that minds are disembodied? Maybe it's cultural? Either way, we're taking a kind of naive and intuitive disembodiment as our starting point and making our way to embodiment from there.

We've tried to make arguments explicit where we can and have included a glossary of technical terms, including some concepts that are a part of logic and critical thinking.

We have found this project enjoyable and enriching. We hope you do too.

For instructors

To start, we want to identify our pedagogical debt to Aristotle. He would often begin his analyses with common opinions and ideas. We do the same kind of thing, beginning with the slogan "mind over matter" as a way of getting into thinking about embodiment. Aristotle also moved between empirical research and philosophical speculation; an Aristotelian approach to doing philosophy is to be conversant with the sciences. We do this too. While this is undoubtedly a *philosophy* book, you'll find plenty of neuroscience, social psychology, and anthropology. Finally, Aristotle famously says in the *Metaphysics* (echoing Plato in the *Theaetetus*) that philosophy begins in wonder. The sense of wonder inspiring us comes from the mind being not only something natural but also something very special. Humans are a part of the natural world, but we're the only species (as far as we know) with complicated grammar, weird kinks, and niche hobbies. Our technologies have evolved over time, and we've evolved with them. Culture informs our worries and concerns, but there are some ways of understanding the world that seem to transcend culture. Are mind and body separate things? Are we embodied minds? Are we "enminded" bodies?[4]

Our first pedagogical commitment is accessibility and engagement, which shapes how we organize and present the material. We have tried to write in a breezy, engaging style with enough bad jokes to keep things manageable. While we both contributed to the writing of the book, there are times when each of us draws on personal experience; we use our initials to indicate who the "I" refers to. We also aim to use examples that resonate with undergraduates. As a result, our examples reflect a bias toward American culture, though we hope they resonate with readers from other cultures as well.

In terms of content, we begin by motivating why students should be concerned with the relationship between mind and body. We use this as a way of introducing disembodiment, which we take to include not only substance dualism but nearly any view that treats minds and bodies as describable in fundamentally distinct vocabularies.. We present disembodiment first because we have found in our experience that it's an intuitive view of the mind for American undergraduates.[5] We then raise problems for disembodied views of mind that point toward embodiment a more promising family of positions. From there, we pivot to Clark and Chalmers's views on the extended mind. We do this because we've have found that very few undergrads—or professionals—are neutral about it. Some love it; some loathe it; but a few are undecided.

We use the extended mind to develop a framework for characterizing different views about embodiment. We group together the various "e's"—embodied, embedded, enactive, extended—as forms of embodiment, emphasizing that their diversity stems from highlighting different aspects of our embodied condition. We take this approach because (1) bracketing some subdivisions in the 4E literature presents embodied cognition as a more unified thesis about the nature of mind, and (2) deploying the technical distinctions too early can hinder more than help newcomers. We present weak embodiment as described by Alvin Goldman in a several places.

We also present strong embodiment as developed by JJ Gibson, Eleanor Rosch, Evan Thompson, Hanne de Jaegher, and Shaun Gallagher, among others. After each presentation, we raise objections.

Once we have the core concepts of embodiment on the table, we turn to applications in free will, ethics, and technology. We do this to show students that embodied cognition and its implications are not confined to theories about the mind. Adopting an embodied view can reshape how we approach a wide range of philosophical issues.

You might notice that we ocassionally present ideas in deliberately stark terms. For example, when we talk about "mind over matter," we interpret it as the claim that the workings of the mind are unconstrained by the body. Does everyone who uses this slogan mean this? Surely not. (Though, just as surely, some do.) We offer these sharpened versions in order to stake out positions clearly. We set aside many subtleties to make the broader landscape easier to see. Our main goal is to give readers a sense of that, which requires striking the right level of detail: too little, and the views become caricatures; too much, and readers lose the forest for the tress. Whenever we employ this kind of exaggeration, we'll note it in the footnotes. We take comfort in Wittgenstein's ladder metaphor–that the reader is to "throw away the ladder after he has climbed up it."[6] After developing the conceptual tools needed to think carefully about embodiment, readers can revisit the simplified versions, see their limits, and move toward more nuanced reflection.

Notes

1 At times, we may even use different "e" terms to talk about this concept (e.g., embodied, extended, embedded, enactive). Though there are interesting distinctions between these terms, we're going to start out with a central view that ties all of these "e"s together. So for now, you can think about these interchangeably.

2 Ben Shuman (in conversation) mentioned that there are a lot of references to *The Simpsons*, suggesting that this book is *actually* for people born in the 1980s and 1990s.

3 See, for example, Trnka and Lorencova (2022).

4 For **St. Thomas Aquinas** (and Aristotle), humans are "ensouled bodies"; that is, we are bodies that are animate. See *Summa Theologica*, Part I, Question 75, Article 4.

5 We hesitate to say "undergraduates" without the national qualifier because, as research in psychology has strongly suggested, undergraduates are not a uniform population across the world. See Nisbett (2003) for an introduction to this research. For similar reasons, we will add the qualifier "American" where necessary. Not being native to other cultures, we're not sure what will resonate with readers, but we hope that the framing is enough to generate some of your own examples if ours don't do it for you.

6 *Tractatus Logico-Philosophicus* §6.54

GRATITUDE

I (CL) read a book one time that had a "Gratitude" section rather than an "Acknowledgment" section. The author explained they wanted to thank, and not merely recognize, all those who had helped along the way. I like this idea and am yoinking it.

CL: There are many people who helped with this book in many ways. Students in my summer 2022, 2023, 2024, and 2025 sections of *Philosophy of Human Nature* were among the early readers and offered feedback that helped make the book more student-friendly. Students in my Fall 2024 class, Embodied Cognition, saw a version that was a bit more developed and offered their thoughts on how to improve it. Thanks to all these students for sharing their thoughts and impressions.

I am grateful to Erik Inglis and Avalyn Renee, who were instrumental in researching and talking through the ideas on embodiment and free will in Chapter 12. I am thankful for Hailey O'Hara, whose discussions and work in an independent study helped form material in the section on embodiment and mental health in Chapter 15. Sophie Brotman has been a wonderful conversation partner around embodiment.

Many thanks to Brooklyn Velora, who helped me to think about embodiment in ways I had not previously considered. I am grateful for her time, care, and generosity of spirit. Garland Rossman likewise helped me think through a range of issues concerning body and mind. I'm grateful for her thoughtfulness and patience in thinking through complex issues.

Thanks to Ben Shuman, who was a generous reader and offered helpful feedback on early drafts. Thank you to John Sutton for his encouragement and support of the project. An anonymous reviewer for Routledge provided extraordinarily supportive and critical feedback on the proposal as well as the first complete draft of the manuscript. This book is much improved as a result. I'm grateful to Katerina Kamprani for permission to use the image of "The Uncomfortable Broom" in §9.4.3.4. Thanks also to our editors, Andy Beck and Phoebe Oliver, for their support and encouragement of the project. They have also been *incredibly* patient.

Finally, my personal debts: Thanks to Nathan Ballantyne, Joe Vukov, Adrian Alsmith, Anna Marie Medina, Mark Ornelas, Tim Weidel, Sou Lee, Sarah Bratt, and Erin Schmidt for support. Anne and Jim Diamond; Margaret and Clint Albaugh; Jes Caulkins and Jeff Bonar; Brian Donahue and Tracey McHenry; Butch and Terre Clossey; Brian Clossey and Ellen Mulligan; and Kate, Clare, and Camila Lassiter are all family members who inquired and encouraged. Maria Howard, Greta LaFore, Pete Diamond, and Danielle Shuman are wonderful and encouraging friends who buoyed my spirits at crucial moments. Finally, my wife Michele and daughters Abigail and Lillian have been a font of love, patience, and support. Words cannot express how much they mean to me and how much their encouragement has sustained me. I could not have completed my parts of the book without them. I dedicate this book to them.

I (AK) didn't encounter a book with a "Gratitude" section, but I find the distinction fitting. What follows is less a catalog of credits than an expression of gratitude. There are simply too many people to acknowledge properly. So many helped me think, shape ideas, and work through problems that it would be easy—if not inevitable—to take their contributions for granted. In many cases, their reliability and generosity were such that they became part of how I thought—temporarily absorbed into the extended system that is/was "AK." I am grateful for this kind of thinking-with, which has been invaluable to my work.

My gratitude includes Adrian Alsmith, along with many philosophically inclined and deeply inspiring people I've had the privilege to work with in industry—what I think of as "philosophers in tech." These include Jess Holbrook, Josh Lovejoy, Benny Croisier, Corbin Cunningham, Chelsea Fleming, Octavio Medina, Allen Bevans, Alexander Reese, Adrien Baranes, Jamie Taylor, Johnny Søraker, and the broader Philosophers at Google community. Their ideas, questions, and standards of thought continue to shape how I see and work.

Finally, this book is offered in gratitude to my wife, Britt, my son, Asher, and my parents—who are not merely acknowledged here, but are, and will always be, part of my mind.

PART 1

Framing the question

1

INTRODUCTION

1.1 Chapter overview

In this chapter, we introduce a bunch of examples for thinking about how mind and body might be related to one another. We begin with an assumption common for many Westerners: mind and body are distinct entities. (You'll see by the end of Chapter 3 that this distinction runs into a lot of difficulties.) We'll see that we have good reasons to think that the slogan "mind over matter" is true. But we'll also have lots of examples for how "matter over mind" is true. We'll round things out by explaining why getting straight to these issues matters for newcomers to philosophy as well as veterans of philosophical reflection.

1.2 Getting into it

I (AK) have just 10 more seconds to go, but it feels like my legs are going to give out. My fitness app is telling me that I've got a few more reps left. Motivated by club records in my headphones, I tell myself: I can do this. I can knock out a few more reps before I'm allowed to stop. What's that expression? "Mind over matter?" Yes. I'm trying to do whatever that thing is. Use my mind, through sheer force of will, to "command" or "make" my body do these reps it's struggling to do. But does this really work for us?

The short answer is: sometimes. We can perform great physical feats, pushing our body beyond its limits through the power of our mind. We hear stories like this all the time: parents lifting cars to save their kids in emergencies, activists going weeks without food or water in protest. Maybe

DOI: 10.4324/9781003356622-2

the mind does "rule" the body. Maybe you can accomplish nearly anything if you set your mind to it.

But if you've got a broken hand, you can't exactly "mind over matter" when writing an essay. If your blood sugar is below 54mg/dl, I doubt you can keep from passing out. Want to will yourself to stay awake forever because sleep is for the weak? I doubt you can...at least not without amphetamines, which only delay the inevitable. There is a breaking point–where physiological constraints override conscious control.[1]

The expression "mind over matter" suggests that *through mental activity, you can overcome bodily limitations*. But, like most common expressions, this is only sort of true some of the time.

> **Otto's workbook**: List 3 times when you wanted to "mind over matter" something, but it didn't work. Why do you think it failed?

Despite all the examples we have that "mind over matter" isn't always true, the idea that the mind is unconstrained by the body is everywhere. It's obvious if you've ever been part of a fitness or dieting group that tries to beat you over the head with the message that it's just a matter of willpower to get the physique you want. Or if you've ever heard that someone can get over addictions if they try hard enough. Troy McClure gives us some useful advice along these lines: "You might remember me from such self-help videos as, *Smoke Yourself Thin* and *Get Confident, Stupid!*"[2]

OK, so if the mind doesn't rule the body all the time, how do we work? Let's consider the alternative: that the body controls the mind.

When I (CL) am hungry, I can be a real jerk. I'm irritable, mean, and just want to get through whatever's between me and food. But I don't want to be an irritable grump. I don't mean to be mean to the people I love. I really *do* want to know about how your day was and look at different paint chips for the living room, but holy guacamole, do I need a burrito. In this case, my body is messing up my mind. I'm hungry or, to be more specific, "hangry." Hanger plagues my existence. Thankfully, those who know me usually recognize this and tell me to get some food. To some extent, we can all relate to being hangry; this is a case of matter over mind.

Same thing goes when I don't sleep well, say, from staying up late partying or lying in bed filled with existential dread about the state of the world (or the amount of stuff I've got to do tomorrow). When this happens, I'm going to be a jerk during the day. I don't want to be a jerk; I only got three hours of sleep. Sorry, I can't help it. Despite the fact that I really, *really* want to be nice to you and pay attention to what you're saying, I'm checked out. It's my body's fault, right? Matter over mind.

Same for people with chronic illness or pain. I don't want to be a jerk, but I feel like I've got a never-ending migraine. It's hard to be patient or sympathetic when I feel like I have a drill boring through my skull.

> **Otto's workbook**: Think about 3 times your body "made" you do something. You wanted to behave or believe in a certain way, but your body said otherwise. What happened? What are some reasons for this?

While the expression "matter over mind" isn't as popular, we can see that it's no more or less true than its opposite. It's kind of true sometimes, and there are lots of times when it's not true.

So what the heck are we? Matter with minds? Minds with some matter? Both views are only "kind of" correct; they get some things right, but also plenty of things wrong.

1.3 Cool story. Who cares?

If you're like we were as college students, you might be wondering why this matters. We'll be asking that question a lot in the last few chapters of the book, but we want to start out with a few motivating cases that are commonplace in American culture.

1.3.1 As many hours in the day as Beyonce (or Bill Gates or...)

You have 24 hours in the day. So do the world's most successful artists and entrepreneurs. So did history's most accomplished figures. What's your excuse?

This kind of thinking has "mind over matter" in the background: You might be as successful as Beyonce (or whoever) if only you would just put your mind to it. The only thing that really matters is your own willpower, your bodily state and environment don't. But if we have reason to doubt "mind over matter," which we do, then this kind of toxic motivational thinking goes the way of the dinosaurs.

Maybe you have some room in your life for more motivation. Maybe you really can do more with your day. But just because Beyonce has accomplished what she has with the same hours in a day as you doesn't mean you're coming up short.

1.3.2 *Cleansing diets*

Detox diets have been all the rage in the US since at least the late 20th century. They typically require a period of restricted consumption: drinking lemon water with cayenne and eating only red meat. After a period of time (3 days, 7 days, 2 weeks, etc.), you'll have cleansed all the "toxins" from your body (whatever those are). You'll have lost weight, and you'll feel better and even think more clearly. Jeffrey Morrison's *Cleanse Your Body, Clear Your Mind* advertises that proper eating can "jump-start" your body's natural detoxification system, which brings with it greater degrees of health and eliminates brain fog.

This is "matter over mind" kind of thinking: all you have to do is get your body into the right state, and you'll feel and think better. All you need to do to improve your mental life is eat the right kinds of things.

Of course, there are foods that help us feel better (kale, apples) and help us feel worse (beer, greasy hamburgers). Eating a balanced diet (whatever that looks like for you) is important to long-term goals like heart health. Maybe you *do* need to drink more water. Or maybe you *do* feel better after a cleansing diet—that's great! But don't confuse that experience with the belief that you *must* get your body into a particular state in order to think clearly.

1.3.3 *And your point is...*

The point of these two examples is to show how we understand the relationship between mind and body affects our lives. If you're the "willpower and gumption" type, but find yourself exhausted at the end of the day, maybe cut yourself a little slack. You have as many hours in the day as Beyonce, but you and she are different people. Maybe she has more self-discipline than you, or maybe not. Maybe she has more money and resources than you, or maybe not. Either way, what comes to mind as important in thinking about your own life depends on how you think the body and mind affect one another.

Let's go from confusion about minds and bodies to doing some philosophy. That's what we're up to in the next chapter.

Notes

1 If you've consumed any laxative with at least 5 mg of Bisacodyl, you'll need to stay near a toilet no matter how strong your willpower or sphincteral fortitude.
2 *The Simpsons*, "Bart's Inner Child," Season 5, Episode 7.

2

FROM APORIA TO PHILOSOPHY

2.1 Chapter overview

We have two conflicting views that leave us feeling unsettled: mind-over-matter and matter-over-mind. To make sense of this tension, we do some philosophy. First, we get clear on what these claims are actually saying: the slogans are ambiguous, and an important part of doing philosophy is clarifying key concepts. Next, we look at different ways of combining the claims and test them for problems. Despite our best efforts, difficulties arise at every turn. We then introduce one final move: identifying a common assumption underlying both views and examining reasons to reject it.

2.2 Enter Aporia

In the introduction, we saw some examples that individually seem ok but as a whole cause confusion. We have some good reason to think it's "mind over matter"—that the body is "ruled over" by the mind. But we also saw that "matter over mind" is a real possibility. So which is it—mind over matter or matter over mind? Maybe both? Or neither? It seems like one or the other *has* to be true, right?

We live with **contradictions** every day. I want to run a marathon, but the couch sure is a lot comfier and less sweaty. You want to be a better musician, but you can't make the time for it. These aren't a huge deal—they're tolerable contradictions.[1] But when we're thinking about heavier stuff, like the nature of mind, we want to make some sense of it all—unresolved tensions are unsatisfying.

DOI: 10.4324/9781003356622-3

The more you know: Turns out, thinking about unresolved tensions as unsatisfying is related to culture. Western cultures (Canada, America, France, Germany, etc.) tend to resist these kinds of contradictions, due in large part to a shared philosophical heritage. East Asian cultures (China, Japan, Taiwan, Vietnam, etc.) tend to be more tolerant of contradictions. Western philosophy takes a cue from Aristotle, who said that nothing can be true *and* false, an idea called the **Principle of Noncontradiction**. Eastern philosophy has **Daoism**, with claims like, "the Tao takes no action, and yet nothing is left undone." A great place to start reading up on these issues is Richard Nisbett's *The Geography of Thought*.

First things first: What does it mean "to make sense of it all"? Consider someone who tells you they're vegetarian, but then you spot them eating a bacon cheeseburger. We try to "make sense" of this information. We take these seemingly contradictory facts and try to make them consistent with one another.[2]

Otto's workbook: Try to come up with three ways to make sense of these two facts: (a) Jane says she's a vegetarian and (b) you saw Jane eat a bacon cheeseburger.

Philosophers want to make sense of facts that don't seem to fit with one another. When facts don't quite line up, it's often a cue that there's something worth thinking through. This is part of doing philosophy: we try to find ways of making sense of the world. By introducing contradictory examples that seem plausible, we're compelled to think about any assumptions going into our discussions. In the case of Jane, the Vegetarian, and her cheeseburgers, you might have assumptions like: vegetarians cannot under any circumstances eat meat and still be vegetarian, so Jane has abandoned her veggie ways. Or maybe: you thought the person was Jane, but it was actually her twin sister Janet, who is a fan of bacon cheeseburgers. When we're doing philosophy, we're put into situations where we have to think harder about some of our basic assumptions.

Being a hypocrite or holding conflicting/contradictory views at the same time, is not a great feeling. Most of us find it deeply unsettling–and for good reason. But when that discomfort shows up, something interesting is often happening. You're growing, learning, and on the verge of enriching your understanding. It doesn't always make the experience feel better, but it *is* a green flag: you may be about to discover something important. Philosophers, for the most part, have a fondness for this feeling. It's where we do our best work and where we tend to thrive. The Greeks had a great word for it: *aporia*.

Aporia comes from the Greek and is often used to mean a kind of paradox or confused state. A lot of **Plato**'s dialogues, for instance, end with *aporia*: participants don't have an answer but are just kind of confused because they're left with a bunch of different and contradictory facts about a thing. But it's not confusion for confusion's sake. Rather, being in a state of *aporia* can help pave the way for better philosophical reflection. With all of the examples on the table—some of them contradictory—we're encouraged to let go of our assumptions. When we asked you to think about Jane, we tried to induce a (mild) state of *aporia*.

We find ourselves in a state of *aporia* with respect to mind and body. We have reasons to think that the mind is independent of the body—that the body isn't essential to any of its operations. But we also have reasons to think that the mind is dependent on the body, that much of our mental life is controlled by our bodily states. At this point, we hope you're a little bit confused in thinking about these examples—does the mind "control" the body or does the body "control" the mind? Which way does the causal influence go: mind to body or body to mind? Or both? Or neither?

We're going to introduce a few tools for getting some clarity. The first tool is to look at various ways of combining two positions. The other tool is to see if the two positions have something in common.

2.3 Possibilities

We have two positions: mind-over-matter and matter-over-mind. We've described these as one taking charge over the other. This isn't clear enough for philosophical speculation for many reasons, including (but not limited to) the ambiguity in "taking charge" and the fact that it doesn't connect in obvious ways with things we want to understand, like causes of and explanations for behavior. Let's sharpen up these positions just a little bit. As you'll see throughout this book, a lot of philosophy is trying to get clear on the questions we're trying to ask.

We said in the previous chapter that "mind-over-matter" means something like "I can overcome bodily limitations by sheer willpower." Let's think about this in terms of explanations: when we explain some bit of behavior by "mind-over-matter," what kind of an explanation are we giving? Here is a plausible interpretation: the person accomplished that behavior by ignoring their bodily states and relying on their willpower.[3] In other words, the explanation for that behavior involves psychological states and processes. When you pass on that slice of pizza because you know it'll be bad news for your digestive system, you are exercising your willpower to overcome your hunger. We explain your resisting the temptation of pizza by pointing to your beliefs and desires, that is, to your mental states. Our new interpretation of mind-over-matter is "explanations for behavior require using the language of psychology."

We can do the same kind of thing for "matter-over-mind." That means something like "bodily capacities overwhelm the best of intentions." We're going to interpret that to mean: "behaviors are explained by bodily states." When you succumb to the temptation of pizza, we can talk about stimulation of your senses and the bodily states associated with that stimulation. So answering the question "why did Giuseppe eat the pizza?" would involve appealing to his visual and olfactory senses and hunger pangs in his stomach.

Let's abbreviate these: MIND will be our shorthand for "explaining behaviors requires appealing to mental or psychological states." MATTER will mean "explaining behaviors requires appealing to bodily states."

For each of MIND and MATTER, it could be true, or it could be false. This gives us four options:

1 MIND and MATTER are both true: mind and body are both relevant for explaining behavior;
2 MIND is true and MATTER is false: behaviors have mental causes; physical causes aren't relevant to explain what's happening;
3 MIND is false and MATTER is true: behaviors have physical causes; mental causes aren't relevant to explain what's happening;
4 MIND and MATTER are both false: there aren't *really* mental or bodily influences; whether there really are minds and bodies isn't all that important.

It'll be helpful to visualize the possibilities. First, we'll show you how it's done with a tasty example. Imagine you have a (vegetarian) burger patty, some bread, and cheese in your fridge. The bread will be part of every option. So what food combinations are possible? (Table 2.1)

Given your ingredients and your commitment to using the bread, you have four choices available to you.

Now consider an example of some mundane behavior. I (CL) drink *a lot* of coffee. You see me one morning leaving my desk and going to the coffee maker to pour a cup of coffee. You could explain this in a few ways. You might point to my crippling caffeine addiction and the ways that my brain and body change as a result of consuming coffee. That is, you could explain my behavior in terms of my biology. On the other hand, you might say

TABLE 2.1 Meat and cheese truth table

		Cheese	
		Yes	*No*
Meat	*Yes*	Burger, cheese (Cheeseburger)	Burger, no cheese (Burger)
	No	No burger, cheese (Grilled Cheese)	No burger, no cheese (Bread sandwich)

TABLE 2.2 Our options for explaining behaviors

		MIND	
		Yes	*No*
MATTER	*Yes*	**Need both.** Have to explain things in terms of both biology and psychology.	**Need only Matter.** Explanation is provided by biology; psychology isn't part of the explanation.
	No	**Need only Mind.** Explanation is provided by psychology; biology isn't part of the explanation.	**No mind and no matter.** Neither biology nor psychology is needed for explanations of behavior.

that Charlie wants coffee, and his wanting explains why he's pouring himself a fifth cup. That is, you could explain my behavior in terms of my psychology.

Let's connect our simple example with our two positions, MIND and MATTER. We want to know our options when we're figuring out what is relevant in explaining behaviors.

There are two "kinds" of information that we can use to explain what's going on. Do we need one or the other? Or do we need both? (Table 2.2).

Philosophers often refer to this kind of exercise as finding the **space of possibilities**. By this, they mean the set of theories (or ideas) that remain after systematically considering different combinations, typically guided by principles of logic. The logical principle at work right now is that all claims are either true or false. (the **Principle of Bivalence.**) One advantage of this approach is that it forces us to consider every option on the table. In doing so, it often prompts us to reconsider our assumptions. Let's take a quick look at each position in the grid and some of the problems they face.

2.3.1 *Mind and matter*

Both psychology and biology matter for an explanation of behavior. One version of this is **identity theory.** Identity theory says that mental states are identical to brain states. Your belief that rocks repel bears[4] is identical to some state of your brain.

Now, when we say "identical," we mean something very specific. To say that two things are identical is to say that we have one thing, but it goes by two different names. This is called "numerical identity." The word "eleven," the Arabic numeral "11," and the Roman numeral "XI" don't pick out different things. There are different ways of referring to the same thing—the number 11. Similarly, "Selina Kyle" and "Catwoman" refer to the same person in the *Batman* comics. "Mark Twain" and "Samuel Clemens" refer to the same person. In this sense, "belief that rocks repel bears" and "brain state B" (where this is some state of the brain) refer to the same thing, the physical brain in a particular state.[5] Some piece of behavior will have both psychological and neurological explanations. One goal of identity theory is to identify **bridge laws** that will enable connections among psychological and neuroscientific explanations.

A common criticism of identity theory is that it appears to deny mental states to anything without a human brain. For example, chimpanzees' brains differ from ours in many crucial respects. Even so, they experience pain. But if being in pain is identical to a brain state, and brain states in chimpanzees differ from those in humans, then chimpanzee pain must differ from human pain. The argument is:

1 Human pain = human brain state B;
2 Chimp pain = chimp brain state B;
3 Human brain state B ≠ chimp brain state B;
4 Therefore, human pain ≠ chimp pain (from 1 to 3 by substitution of identicals).

But the conclusion seems a kind of odd. Humans and chimps exhibit many of the same pain behaviors, like screaming and avoidance behaviors. In fact, it's intuitive to think that chimps experience pain like we do *because* they exhibit the same kinds of behaviors.

2.3.2 *No mind but matter*

Psychology doesn't matter as part of an explanation of behavior; only neuroscience does. This view – known as **eliminativism** – holds that there are no such things as minds. Neuroscience will tell us everything we need to know about thinking and consciousness. This was developed and popularized by **Paul** and **Patricia Churchland**. Whenever we're talking about the mind, we're using inaccurate language. It might be useful, but it's not true. A good analogy is how we talk about the sun "rising" or "setting." The sun isn't doing either of these things: the Earth is rotating, and the Sun appears to be moving across the sky. Sunsets don't exist, if by that we mean that the Sun *moves* from one horizon to another. In the same way, beliefs and experiences don't exist; it's activity in the brain only that exists. We can talk about beliefs as long as they don't do any harm, but they don't exist. We *eliminate* our theories about mind in favor of theories about brains.

Otto's workbook: Eliminativism about all kinds of things is common in the history of science. For instance, scientists posited the existence of phlogiston to explain combustion. Phlogiston was a gas or fluid that was released when an object burned. When the object was done burning, what was left was the dephlogisticated material. We know now that combustion is a process where a substance is rapidly combined with oxygen to produce light and heat. Once chemists discovered what combustion really is, they got rid of the concept of phlogiston. Do you think all our mental concepts will go the way of phlogiston? Suppose they do; what would that mean for how we think about mental health or explanation our behavior?

One problem often cited for eliminativism is that we can't abandon our mental concepts. We describe and explain human behavior using mental concepts, and doing so is useful. When the courts punish someone for theft, they rely on many terms connected to our ideas about the mind: the person *intended* to break in; they were not *apologetic* about doing it; they were *aware* that their actions were illegal; they *knew* the consequences of being caught and *believed* they would escape. Now imagine what these descriptions would look like if we replaced all the mental language with talk about brains. What would make those neural descriptions meaningful are the very mental concepts eliminativism asks us to discard. We can't get away from them, even if we tried.

2.3.3 Mind but no matter

What matters in an explanation of behaviors is psychology, not biology or neuroscience. This position is known as **functionalism** (and we'll have much more to say about it in Chapter 3). According to functionalism, minds are input-output systems: they *take in* perception and thoughts and *produce* thoughts and actions. Individual mental states are defined by these roles–by what causes them (their inputs) and what they in turn cause (their outputs).

Take pain. Pain is a state that is caused by stubbing your toe (among other things) and that can cause swearing and grunting (among other things). That functional role is all there is to being in pain. Crucially, functionalism holds that we can describe mental states entirely in these terms, without any reference to the physical stuff the thinking thing is made of. The underlying material simply doesn't matter. It might be biological, but it could just as well be mechanical or alien. In principle, any kind of material can realize mental states.

On this view, mental states are what matter for explaining behavior. Bodily states do not. They are merely the *vehicles* that realize mental states. Of course, minds don't float freely around the world like ghosts—you need some physical substrate—but for functionalists, that substrate plays no explanatory role. What does the explaining are the mental states themselves.

Ned Block offers a famous objection to functionalism. Suppose functionalism turns out to be right. If the matter really doesn't matter, we can imagine the nation of China as a single, thinking organism. How? In 2021, there were roughly 1.5 billion Chinese citizens. Imagine each citizen is given a switch that controls whether a silicon chip in a robot is on or off—much like how the neurons in our brain either fire or do not. Now imagine that these citizens, watching their TVs, are given a signal whether to turn their switch on or off. Everyone in Beijing turns their switches on, while everyone in the Sichuan province turns them off. The citizens of China would be the "brain" of the robot: all control would come from the coordinated efforts of the citizens. But this seems weird: how could a country of people be a mind? So, Block argues that functionalism is *too permissive*. It allows too many things to count as having minds. As we're going to see, the functionalist idea of inputs and outputs is going to give us the ingredients for extended mind.

2.3.4 No mind and no matter

Neither psychology nor biology is needed for our explanations. What then might be required? There are different ways you can run with this. Here are a few.

2.3.4.1 Physics is all you need

It might be that you only need physics: the world is made up of atoms and so physics will ultimately provide explanations of behavior. At some point *way* in the future, psychology will be understood in terms of biology. Biology will be understood in terms of chemistry. Chemistry will be understood in terms of physics. So explanations of behavior will be given by the physicists.

The concern with this notion is parallel to that of eliminativism: behavior given in terms of atoms is meaningful to us because of our psychological explanations. Suppose you were to explain some behavior in terms of positions of atomic particles: atoms numbered 1–12,300 move in *this* direction, while atoms numbered 12,301–50,026 move over *there*, and atoms numbered… What's happened? What transpired? Did someone eat a sandwich? Steal a candy bar? Save a kitten? The significance of the behavior described in terms of atoms wouldn't be obvious unless you connected it with beliefs, desires, and intentions.

2.3.4.2 Anthropology is all you need

Maybe, though, we're just pawns being pushed around the chess game of life. We do what we do because of social and cultural programming. I (CL) don't like to eat bugs because my American cultural upbringing has shaped me in a way to prefer a certain range of foods, which does not include insects. Anthropologists work on identifying the sociocultural laws and principles that govern our behavior. So explanations of behavior will be given by the anthropologists.

The worry for this view is that human behavior would no longer be explained in terms of choices or internal states. You might think you dislike fried grasshoppers because the idea disgusts you, but on this view that reaction is really a product of cultural conditioning. You might think it's wrong to steal from others because you hold beliefs about property rights, but those beliefs, too, would be traced back to cultural forces. While this position is not logically inconsistent, accepting it would require a significant reworking of many of our core concepts—free will, responsibility, morality, and politics, to name just a few.

2.3.4.3 Effective predictions are all you need

Daniel Dennett develops instrumentalism, which holds that it doesn't ultimately matter whether minds really exist. What matters is whether treating something as if it has a mind helps us understand and predict its behavior. For example, if we see you making a sandwich while salivating, we can anticipate what you'll do next by interpreting you as hungry and as believing that eating the sandwich will satisfy that hunger.

Contrast this with a coffee maker. It doesn't hold beliefs about the world, nor does it want or fear anything. Treating it as if it had a mind would add nothing to our ability to explain or predict what it does. From an instrumentalist perspective, then, we need not settle whether behavior is driven by mental states or bodily states in any deep metaphysical sense. What matters is simply whether adopting the language of mental states helps us make sense of what's going on.

One criticism of such a view is that it leaves open a huge gap in explaining human behavior. We know that concepts like "belief" and "intention" are useful for explaining and predicting human behavior. For example, if Mika is turning the key in the ignition, she *believes* that the car will start and she *intends* to start the car. But if there really aren't beliefs and desires (or if we're neutral about whether they exist or not), then why is treating Mika like she has beliefs and intentions so useful? **Jerry Fodor** offered this concern.

We've uncovered something important: every possible combination of mind and matter leads to difficulties. That's a strong clue that a deeper problem is at work.

2.4 What MIND and MATTER have in common

We've laid out the space of possibilities for MIND and MATTER. But is that all there is? Are there more philosophical moves to make?

Indeed, there are. When two positions *seem* opposed—or can be reconciled only by restricting them to different cases or contexts— we look for what they share in common. And if they do share something, we can then ask whether we have good reason to accept it.

> **Otto's workbook**: Imagine you and a friend are deciding what to do for dinner in a small town with only a few places to eat. Your friend says, "Look, our options tonight are Olive Garden or Red Lobster." What assumption is your friend making about your dinner options? More specifically, what assumption would you have to challenge in order to say, "We don't have to do either of those"?

At first, it might seem absurd to assume that MIND and MATTER have anything in common. After all, one view says the mind is "in charge of" the body, while the other says the body is "in charge of" the mind. But what these views share is how they set up the problem in the first place.

Both treat mind and body as opposed—or at least distinct—entities: mind *versus* body, or mind *and* body conceived as two separate things. Much of the philosophy of mind over the past few centuries has been devoted to solving the **mind–body problem**: explaining how the mind and body are connected. But for there to be a "mind–body problem" at all, minds and bodies must first be treated as the kinds of things that require a story about how they connect.

That brings us to two tasks. First, we need to clarify what this way of setting up the problem involves. Second, we need to show why it's worth questioning. We begin that work by examining **disembodiment**, which is the focus of the next chapter.

Notes

1 Strictly speaking, these aren't contradictions; they are tensions. A contradiction is asserting that *p* and *not-p* are both true, like "grass is green" and "grass is not green" at the same time. A contradiction is always false. In contrast, a **tautology** is always true, like "grass is green or it is not green."

2 Philosophers call this process, achieving **reflective equilibrium**. The goal is to strike a balance among different—and potentially inconsistent—pieces of information, as well as general rules for thinking. **Nelson Goodman** in his book *Fact, Fiction, and Forecast* is often credited for bringing the concept to the attention of contemporary readers and philosophers.

3 This approach has roots in Aristotle. In his works on metaphysics and the natural world, he introduces four causes. These are sometimes better understood as four "becauses" (Jaworski 2011). They are answers to "why?" questions. For Aristotle and other philosophers, the line between causes and explanations is blurry. **Elizabeth Anscombe** adopts a similar approach in her book *Intention*, where she says that intentions are answers to "why" questions. By taking this approach, we can remain neutral on what causes what and instead focus on explaining how one thing brings about another. Are minds real? Do they causally affect the world or is it really the brain? We don't have answers to these questions, but we use mental language to explain why people do what they do. By thinking about explanations instead of (say) causes, we can avoid tough questions about the reality of mind and focus on how we explain things in the world.

4 Cf. *The Simpsons*, "Much Apu About Nothing," season 7 episode 23.

5 **Gottlob Frege**, often credited with being one of the founding figures of contemporary analytic philosophy, was interested in puzzles about identity like these. He noted that "the Morning Star" and "the Evening Star" were both expressions used by the ancient Greeks to refer to the same thing—namely, the planet Venus. And while "the Morning Star is the Morning Star" is trivially true (that is, it is as informative as saying "Venus is Venus"), "the Morning Star is the Evening Star" was an important empirical discovery, even though both sentences are made true by the same situation! **Saul Kripke**, in the landmark book *Naming and Necessity*, draws some fascinating connections between identity theory and Frege's puzzles about identity in order to criticize identity theory.

3

THE RISE AND FALL OF DISEMBODIMENT

3.1 Chapter overview

Disembodiment is a claim about the nature of the mind. It says that the mind works independently of the body; or, in other words, that the body is irrelevant to understanding how the mind works. Our previous claims of "mind-over-matter" and "matter-over-mind" both assume that the mind is disembodied. Do we have reason to reject this assumption? Yes. But doing so requires reframing how we think about the nature of the mind. We present some of the basic ideas about mental representations and a computational view of the mind. We begin by presenting these views in stark terms, without qualifications. Later, we complicate the picture and introduce important refinements.

3.2 Disembodiment: the basic idea

> **Otto's workbook**: In 1943, Disney put out a short cartoon called "Reason and Emotion." You should be able to find the roughly 8 minute clip on YouTube. Do you think this more or less accurately portrays the kind of back-and-forth we feel when we're thinking about what we should do? Why or why not?

The film is significant for several reasons. It was produced in part as U.S. propaganda to push back against the emotionally charged rhetoric found in Hitler's speeches. The basic idea is that our capacity to reason can help counteract the kinds of emotions dictators try to stir in their citizens.

DOI: 10.4324/9781003356622-4

Jump ahead 70 years to another Disney film, *Inside Out*. Here, a young girl named Riley moves from Minnesota to California for her dad's job. Viewers get a front-row seat to her emotional life. We see Sadness, Anger, Joy, Fear, and Disgust represented as human-like creatures, guiding Riley's actions. At the movie's climax, Anger has had enough of attempting to fit into her new life and, as a result, Riley attempts to run away to Minnesota.

What these films have in common is that they represent emotions and reason as person-like entities that exist inside our heads. There are lots of other examples in pop culture: *Herman's Head* was a short-lived sitcom where we watched impulses and emotions fight it out over what the titular character, Herman, would do. In *The Simpsons*, you'll often find a voice inside a character's head, addressing the character as though it were a separate person. The film *Being John Malkovich* imagined people crawling through a small door and becoming the person inside of John Malkovich, guiding his actions.

Otto's workbook: Let's drive home just how deeply embedded the concept of disembodiment is in pop culture. Find seven examples of movies, TV shows, or stories that involve body-swapping like *Freaky Friday*. If you really want to challenge yourself, limit your examples to the last ten years.

These movies imagine the mind as something that works independently of the body. In *Inside Out*, for example, Riley's emotions compel her to act, yet they are not anchored to her body in any obvious way. There are levers and buttons that control Riley's behavior, but that is the extent of the mind–body connection depicted. In "Reason and Emotion," we see the faculties of reason and emotion fighting for control, treating the body (literally) as the vehicle they use to get around. These examples reflect the basic idea behind **disembodiment**: that minds work independently of the bodies to which they are attached.

The more you know (*don't skip this one!*): Disembodiment is a claim about how minds *work*. There are stronger and weaker forms of this claim. The *strong* version says that minds *are* independent of bodies, and hence work independently of bodies. This is equivalent to Cartesian dualism: minds and bodies are made of separate substances. They're literally different kinds of things. The *weak* version says that minds may or may not exist independently of bodies, but we can understand how minds work without having to understand anything about bodies. This weak sense of disembodiment is captured by *functionalism*—which you read about in §2.2.3. In philosophy of science, this weak disembodiment is known as the **autonomy of psychology**: psychology is a discipline independent of (and not reducible to) biology and neuroscience. In the metaphysics of mind, weak disembodiment is expressed in **non-reductive physicalism**: the mind is a physical thing, but its operations are not reducible to bodily processes. Throughout this book, we will be using "disembodiment" in the *weak* sense.

Once you notice this, you see disembodiment popping up elsewhere. The key is to find examples where the mind is imagined as working without reference to the body or where the body acts as a vehicle for the mind to get around. Want another example? Here you go: uploading your consciousness onto a computer. If it were possible to do this, then you would no longer be inhabiting a body. Instead, you would be located "in" a machine: your consciousness would be in the silicon chips of a supercomputer instead of the neurons of your brain. If you think this is plausible, then congratulations: you've accepted the premise of disembodiment. And if your consciousness can be uploaded to a computer, then your consciousness doesn't require your *brain* in order to exist. It can't exist free-floating on its own, for sure, but it doesn't require a specific kind of material. Your consciousness can be **realized** in silicon chips or neurons. How consciousness works is independent of the "stuff" that is conscious.

In a lot of ways, disembodiment seems perfectly natural, almost obvious. After all, others don't know what you're thinking or feeling unless you tell them. That is, our thoughts and feelings are private: they aren't available for others. Another way of putting this is that we have **privileged access** to our own thoughts. Each of us occupies a privileged position with respect to our own mental life. We can know what we're thinking, but others don't. These features seem central to our ordinary concept of mind, and disembodiment easily accounts for them. All of this helps explain why disembodiment seems true.

Disembodiment weaves throughout the history of philosophy. You can find it in **Plato**'s description of the soul in the *Phaedo*: he describes the soul as distinct from the body and able to be reincarnated. There's a similar dualist conception found in **St. Augustine**'s work. In the medieval Islamic tradition and influenced by Plato, **Ibn Sina**[1] and **Al-Kindi** are dualists. In modern philosophy, **Rene Descartes** is typically considered the instigator of our current conceptions of mind and body. Descartes is famous for saying,

"I think; therefore, I am." In other words, the fact that you're thinking is indubitable evidence that you exist. (After all, how could you be aware of thinking if you didn't exist to do the thinking?)

What we're most interested in is mind-body dualism. You encountered dualism in Chapter 2. The idea is that there are two kinds of stuff in reality: mental stuff and physical stuff, and neither depends on the existence of the other. Descartes arrives at this conclusion at the end of the *Meditations on First Philosophy*. The argument goes like this:

1 If the mind is the body, then they could never be distinct things;
2 But mind and body *could* be distinct things;
3 Therefore, the mind is not the body.[2]

The argument for premise 1 goes like this. Suppose the mind is the body—for instance, the mind is the brain. Then, one can't exist without the other. Mind and body (or brain) would be like Spiderman and Peter Parker, Mark Twain and Samuel Clemens, Cassius Clay and Muhammad Ali. If you bump into Cassius Clay, then you've bumped into Muhammad Ali. If you high-five Samuel Clemens (awkward because he's dead), then you've given a high-five to Mark Twain. Importantly, whenever you have one member of each pair (Spiderman, Peter Parker; Mark Twain, Samuel Clemens), you have the other. It couldn't possibly be otherwise.

Premise 2 argues, in contrast, that it's possible for the mind to exist without the body. How do we think about what's possible in the broadest sense? Usually, we depend on our imaginations.[3] Could there be a world in which a hobbit named Frodo has to throw a ring into Mount Doom? Sure—JRR Tolkien describes just such a world for us. Or could there be a universe where pigs fly, and chocolate is explosive? Totally. So now, can you imagine a world in which the mind exists independently of the body? Of course you can! Just imagine yourself floating in deep space (pretend that problems like breathing and hypothermia have been taken care of by evolution or magic). Could you have conscious experiences in this case? Could you think to yourself, "I'm thinking?" Sure, you could!

Side quest: Descartes' ideas are foreshadowed in the work of St. Augustine, St. Teresa of Avila, and Ibn Sina. Choose one of these thinkers and read about them in the *Internet Encyclopedia of Philosophy*. For St. Teresa, read the essay, "One of Descartes' most famous ideas was first articulated by a woman," in the online magazine *Quartz*.[4] In what ways are this thinker's view similar to Descartes? In what ways are they different?

This **thought experiment** suggests that it's possible for the mind and the body to exist independently of one another, which is just what premise 2 says. The conclusion follows from the premises by *modus tollens*.

Fast forward roughly 300 years to the 20th century. Disembodiment is still alive and well, but not in the strong form we find in Descartes. It's undergone a transformation in philosophy and cognitive science. Nowadays, disembodiment doesn't mean that the mind is a separate *thing* that can exist apart from the body. Instead, it shows up as the possibility of doing psychology without regard to the body; that is, the body doesn't play an essential role in psychological research.

Otto's workbook: What does it mean to do psychology by talking about the body? This theory, **behaviorism**, focuses on *observable behavior*. Psychology, behaviorists remind us, is the study of human *behavior*. And to study human behavior, we must work only with what is observable—no unobservable entities allowed. So behaviorism prohibited the supposition that there were unobservable, internal processes involved in thinking. To do so would be to go beyond the available data. The study of human behavior therefore meant studying stimuli and responses. One infamous study by the famed behaviorist John Watson was the Little Albert Experiment. Read the entry on the Little Albert Experiment in *Wikipedia*. Summarize it in 150 words. Be sure to identify the stimulus, the response, and how Watson (and other behaviorists) understood the concept of a *phobia*. For extra credit, write 50 words on why scientists should take ethics classes.

A useful jumping-off point for understanding disembodiment in the 20th century is the work of **Alan Turing**. In his paper "*Computing Machinery and Intelligence*," published in 1950, Turing asked, "can machines think?" The test he proposed (now known as the Turing Test) works like this. Put a human judge at a computer terminal. The judge can type questions to two entities: one is a person (also at a computer terminal), and the other is a computer. If the judge can't tell the difference between the person and the computer, then the computer has passed the Turing Test.

Our way into disembodiment begins by examining similarities between humans and computers. This approach has been picked up by philosophers as well as psychologists and neuroscientists, so we're in good company.

3.3 Disembodiment meets science: a primer on mental representations and computations

Disembodiment is still somewhat vague at this point, but it's been made more precise through developments in cognitive science. There are many ways to tell the history of cognitive science.[5] We're going to start with the **Cognitive Revolution** and Alan Turing.[6]

3.3.1 Minds as computers

The Cognitive Revolution is a revolution in the sense that it rejected many of the fundamental ideas of psychology that were mainstream in the USA at the time. The framework in vogue was behaviorism, which said that the only useful data for psychological explanation were overt behavior. Cognitivism (the framework ushered in by the cognitive revolution) posited all manner of internal entities, including mental representations and computational procedures. In essence, cognitivism claims that there *must* be internal, unobservable entities in order to explain human behavior.

The more you know: The linguist **Noam Chomsky** is often credited with ushering in the Cognitive Revolution with his 1959 review of **B.F. Skinner**'s book on language, titled *Verbal Behavior*. Consider, for a moment, how a bird communicates. It produces sounds to identify its territory and to find mates. Birds, by and large, are hardwired to make these kinds of sounds. There is a stimulus—seeing a potential mate—and a behavior, making the appropriate sound. However, birds—pigeons in particular—can be made to respond to certain kinds of stimuli. Skinner performed many experiments in which a pigeon would repeat some bit of behavior if it received food while doing that behavior. If the pigeon bobbed its head and Skinner threw in some food, the pigeon would bob its head again. This kind of learning is called **operant learning**: behaviors are learned through reward and punishment. Skinner's hypothesis was that children learn language through rewards and punishments. A child makes a noise that sounds like "horse" while looking at a horse and the parent praises the child. That same child makes the same sound while looking at a pig and the parent the child.

Chomsky's argument, in brief, is that there is no explicit teaching as children acquire language, something that, Chomsky claims, Skinner's theory would require. One of the key arguments Chomsky offers is the **Poverty of the Stimulus**. The nutshell version of the argument is: kids aren't exposed to enough information in their development to account for their sophisticated language abilities. (That is, there is a *poverty* of *stimuli*.)[7] The best explanation for kids' language abilities (Chomsky argues) is that they have an innate "program" for language that is activated when children are immersed in a linguistic environment.

Some of the ideas of the Cognitive Revolution come from Alan Turing, who described an "imitation game" in his paper "Computing Machinery and Intelligence." He asks us to imagine a questioner sitting at a computer terminal. The questioner inputs questions that go to a machine and to a person. The machine and the person then give their answers, and the questioner must figure out which is the machine and which is the person. This has come to be known as the **Turing Test**. The central idea is: if a machine can answer questions in a way that's indistinguishable from a human's responses, then the machine is intelligent.[8] This is connected to another important essay Turing wrote, "On Computable Numbers, with an Application to the *Entscheidungsproblem*." Don't let the German scare you. *Entscheidungsproblem* means "decision problem." The problem, posed as a question, is: is there a process for determining whether a randomly chosen formula of logic (like, "if person x is tall, then someone is tall") is provable? Turing proves the answer is "no," but more interesting for us is *how* he got there. He describes a kind of machine that can calculate the solution to any mathematical problem that has a solution—this has come to be called a **Turing machine**.[9] A Turing machine has an infinitely long tape and all it can do is erase or print a symbol on this tape and move left or right along the tape. A Turing machine is always in some kind of state, where a state is a description of how the machine is set to behave—kind of like how you're disposed to be grumpy when you're hungry. It also has a set of instructions for what to do. One example of an instruction is, "if you are in state A and you are reading a '1' on the tape, erase the '1', move to the left and go into state B." These machines are the forerunners of the modern computer.

Hilary Putnam, in his paper, "*The Mental Life of Some Machines*," uses Turing's ideas to think about our own minds. Putnam observes that machines' behaviors can be described in terms of "if...then..." statements. Sometimes they're simple: if the dishwasher is running, it will spray water. Sometimes they're a smidge more complicated: if your laptop is on and you have a word processing document open and you push "f", then an "f" will appear on your screen. But at the end of the day, it's all "if...then..." statements. Notice that we can do the same thing for people: if Charlie believes Aaron took the last taco, then Charlie will be sad.

We can even do this for mental states like belief and desire: if Lily sees a turkey in the yard, then she will believe there is a turkey in the yard. If Susan smells cake, then she will want cake.

Otto's workbook: *Part 1*: Come up with three examples of "if...then..." sentences where there's a perception in the "if" part and a belief or desire in the "then" part.

Part 2: Now come up with scenarios for each of them where the "if" part is true and the "then" part is false. For the cake-sniffer example above, it might be that Susan smells the cake but feels nauseous, and so doesn't want the cake—the "if" part is true (she smells the cake) and the "then" part is false (she doesn't want the cake). What do you think this means for describing our behaviors and mental states in terms of "if...then..." sentences?

Machines are described by "if…then…" statements. Human behaviors and mental states are described by "if…then…" statements. What explains the similarity? Putnam suggests that it's the **computational theory of mind.** It says that minds work more or less like computers: minds are the software and brains are the hardware. Just as the circuits in your phone or laptop can represent things about the world—like when you use Google Maps to get from your home to the grocery store—you have **mental representations** you have mental representations that represent things about the world. Your belief that the Earth is round is mentally represented. And any thinking you do can (in principle) be done by a computer: thinking is just rules that can be implemented on a sufficiently powerful computer.

The more you know: Representation is a trigger word for us and lots of other people. It means different things in different circles (e.g., Computer Science, Neuroscience, Linguistics, Philosophy) and people aren't always careful about how they use it. Nevertheless, "representation" often implies theories of mind and perception that make it easier for philosophers to miss the role of the body in cognition.

When AK was an undergraduate, he did a project on face blindness and embodiment. He had both philosophers and psychologists on his committee reviewing his work. Towards the end of the project, each of his committee members began arguing with one another. Things grew heated, and it was almost as if they forgot AK was in the room. What were they arguing about? *Representations*! The specific details aren't important here, but there's a concern worth bringing up.

There's a widespread idea that "perception is a process *in the brain* whereby the perceptual system constructs an *internal representation* of the world"

(Noe 2004). As we explore the world, we transduce sense data through our sense organs (eyes, skin, nose, etc.). Then, we take these data and re-present them in our heads. On the surface, this seems like a reasonable, biologically accurate, causal explanation—one that's consistent with what we know about how our bodies physically work. But here's the problem: who or what are these things re-presented *to*?[10] There are lots of possibilities, but each is as troublesome as the next. It's certainly not some little homunculus[11] in our head, looking at these images. Even if we ignore what kind of entity is looking at the information, we've got to ask: what's it looking at representations with? The "mind's eye"? If so, we've just moved the perceptual "bump in the carpet" further back into our heads. That is, how are *these* re-presentations *perceived*?

Do representations work like "pictures in the mind"? If we answer yes, we run into the problem of an **infinite regress**. Daniel Dennett (1968, 134), in "Nature of Images and the Introspective Trap" sums this point up well when he states:

> For an image to work as an image there must be a person (or an analogue of a person) to see or observe it, to recognize or ascertain the qualities in virtue of which it is an image of something…[but] if we suppose that the product of the perceptual process is an image, we shall have to design a perceiver-analogue to sit in front of the image, and yet another to sit in front of the image which is the end product of perception in the perceiver-analogue and so forth ad infinitum….

You might say, this seems absurd, no one really thinks this is true. And you're right—few, if any, self-respecting professionals in this space actually think that. But if you look at the way "representation" is used in their work or professional discussions, it often seems otherwise.

This doesn't mean that representations always imply mental images and fall victim to the introspective trap. Nor does it mean that representations cannot exist in the mind/brain. It's just that we need to be careful with this concept. We can (and should) use it but we must do so under a paradigm that doesn't imply "inner perception" or mental *images*.

This is just a warning from us. When you come across the term "representation," make sure you've got clarity on what is meant by it. Keep the introspective trap in mind, and avoid it at all costs!

3.3.2 Detail on mental representations: vehicles and contents

Representations are analyzed into two components: their **vehicles** and their **content**. The content is the meaning: it's what the sentences, "the cat is white," "el gato es blanco," "kot jest biały," and "bisadu waa cadaan" have in common. The vehicle is what carries the meaning. For language, the sentences "the cat is white" and "el gato es blanco" carry the meaning that *the cat is white*. The written sentences are the vehicle for that meaning. If I say the sentence, "the cat is white," then my speech is the vehicle for the content that *the cat is white*.

The more you know: Talking about meaning is hard, and writing about it can be even harder. Consider a sentence like, "the cat is white." How do we write what that sentence means? Philosophers (and linguists) often use italics or bold font or all-caps to represent the meaning of the sentence: *the cat is white*. We're going to use italics in this book.

Additionally, I can have the thought "the cat is white" and that thought carries the meaning that *the cat is white* just like the written and spoken sentences. Thoughts, then, have both content and a vehicle: the meaning and what carries it. If you're ever confused about vehicles and their contents, come back to sentences in different languages that mean the same thing. What they mean is the content; the different marks or strings of letters on the page are the vehicles.

Mental representations are information-bearing entities. The process of thinking is (a) storing, (b) changing, and (c) retrieving these entities. So my thought "the cat is white" is a mental representation that carries the information, that *the cat is white*. I might store this information in memory for use at a later date. When I remember it, I'm retrieving it from memory. Sound kind of familiar? Computers store, change, and retrieve information. We do what computers do, just at a level beneath conscious awareness.

Mental representations are **theoretical entities**—this means that scientists suppose they exist and then develop theories and experiments on that supposition. This isn't anything new. When Darwin developed his theory of natural selection, he posited that there was some entity to explain how traits were passed from one generation to the next. We later learned that genes are how that happens. Mental representations are theoretical entities, just like genes were. There's been a lot of research done that assumes their existence. In early 2024, searching for "mental representation" on Google Scholar returned over 400,000 hits. And some of the most famous results in psychology offer explanations in terms of mental representations.[12]

But no philosopher or scientist thinks that if you open up the skull, you're going to see little representations floating around. In the late 20th and early 21st centuries, philosophers, cognitive scientists, and neuroscientists have come to think about mental representations in terms of neurons. A mental representation is often taken to be a convenient way of talking about neural structures in the brain.

The more you know: The scientist **David Marr** worked on vision. In his landmark book—aptly titled *Vision*—he described three levels of explanation for cognitive activity. (We're going to use lingo from **Zenon Pylyshyn** because that's more familiar.) The lowest level is the physical. This is the hardware of the system. For people, it's neurons. For machines, it's silicon chips. Next up, we have the **syntactic** level. This is where we find the structure of mental representations. Remember when we were talking about cats being white? The representation in your head that means *the cat is white* has a syntax (i.e. a grammar) and that's studied at the syntactic level. It might be helpful to think about logical inference. "The cat is white" logically implies "something is white." The logical implication is a result of the structure (or *syntax*) of the representation. Finally, at the highest level, there is the semantic level. This is where we talk about the meaning of representations. When you think about the cat being white, the meaning of that representation (that is, *the cat is white*) is studied at the semantic level. Here, we ask how a mental representation comes to have the meaning that it has and how that meaning gets connected to sentences in a language.

Take, for example, a famous study about **working memory** by the psychologist **George Miller**. He noticed that working memory has a limit. You can only remember so much information before it starts to slip. In a 1956 paper titled "The Magical Number 7, Plus or Minus 2," he argued that working memory—which is the kind of memory we use when we're trying to remember a bit of information to complete a task in the next few seconds or minutes—has a capacity of 7 (plus or minus 2) bits. In this paper, he talked about "information" and "channels," but he didn't talk at all about neurons or neurotransmitters. Since Miller published this paper, there has been a flood of research in neuroscience that has uncovered a wealth of insights into brain activity involved in memory. Miller posited that mental representations have a finite capacity that's measurable in experiments, and neuroscientists have been uncovering the neural structures that make working memory possible.

Now, let's talk about *how* those mental representations are part of mental processes. Computationalism says (very roughly) that those mental representations are manipulated and transformed in ways that a computer could carry out. Take, for instance, the sentence, "Aaron loves Meno the dog." If someone can think this, then they can also think "Meno the dog loves Aaron." A slightly more complicated example involves transforming declarative sentences into questions. For instance, "Charlie is there" can, through the use of rule-governed changes, become "where is Charlie?" Finally, consider that it's possible to embed parts of a sentence within itself, for example, "The boy who is in front of the girl asked for a cookie" can become "the boy who is in front of the girl who is in front of the girl asked for a cookie" and so on. These changes from one sentence to another can be characterized in terms of rules for embedding the same clause inside the sentence over and over again to get new sentences.

These rules can be implemented on a computer. You could easily program a computer to change any sentence of the form "x VERB y" into "y VERB x" (provided the verb is of the right kind—think "loves," not "writes"). Computationalism says that this is what thinking is: changing and storing mental representations in ways that follow rules that a computer could (in theory) implement.

Side quest: Machines using the view of computationalism described above are sometimes called "symbol systems." This is because the representations act as symbols, representing the world. There's another kind of computationalism: **connectionism**. Connectionism conceives of our cognitive system as structured more like our brains. There are lots of connections among nodes and information flows along those connections. You can see this in action at playground.tensorflow.org. Try different combinations of data, features, hidden layers, and neurons. Your goal is to get the "test loss" as close to 0 as possible. As you're playing with those neural networks, ask yourself, "where are the representations?"...or even whether there are representations at all!

One result of the Cognitive Revolution is thinking about minds in terms of mental representations. It's hard to overstate the importance of mental representations in philosophy and psychology. It quickly became a foundational concept much research because it fit quite well with a lot of developments in psychology. For example, remember the example from Chapter 3 about George Miller and the magical number 7 (+/- 2) for the limits of working memory? The limits of working memory are given in terms of how much information the mind can keep in working memory. Information is just another way of describing content! Almost any time you read something in psychology talking about representations or information, you're back in the representationalist paradigm. Representationalism has become (more or less) the default position in psychology and cognitive science.

3.3.3 Intentionality and representations

Thoughts are *about* things. Beliefs about ice cream are about ice cream. Desires for coffee are for coffee. Beliefs, desires, and most mental states are peculiar in this way: they are about things. A belief is always a belief about something; a desire is a desire for something. Philosophers have a term to describe this feature of mental states: they are **intentional** and the general property of interest is **intentionality.**

Intentionality has been taken not just as *a* feature of mental states but as their defining feature. It is often called the "mark of the mental"—a phenomenon counts as mental only if it is intentional. A state is a mental state insofar as it has intentionality. But what's so special about intentionality? There have been oceans of ink spilled on the subject, but we'll keep our discussion brief. In recent history, the discussion is often traced back to **Franz Brentano**. In his book *Psychology from an Empirical Standpoint*, he observes that psychological phenomena are different from physical ones. Most importantly, you can want a sandwich that doesn't exist, but you can't eat a sandwich that doesn't exist. You can imagine a horse with wings, but you'll never ride a horse with wings.

> **Otto's workbook**: Come up with five more examples like the last two. They follow the pattern: "You can [psychological verb] an [object] but you can't [action verb] that [same object]." The aim is to drive home how unusual our mental lives are in this way.

Brentano suggested that the objects of thought have an "intentional inexistence." The lingo sounds odd to our ears (we'll just keep using "intentional"), but it highlights an important idea: *believing* something doesn't make it true and thinking about something doesn't make it real. A big question for philosophers of mind is how to characterize intentional objects: what exactly is an imagined horse? What is the relationship between thought and reality?

One way to make sense of the intentionality of thoughts is to claim that the objects of thought are representations! If you believe "the cat is white," then you have a mental representation that the cat is white.

That representation may or may not correspond to reality. (Maybe the cat is black, or maybe there's no cat at all.) But thinking about the objects of our thoughts as representations gives us a tidy way of understanding intentionality: the intentional objects of our thoughts (i.e., what our beliefs are beliefs about, what our desires are desires for) are mental representations. Since they represent reality (and aren't *actually* reality), believing something doesn't make it true. To say "John believes that coffee makes life worth living" is to say something about John and the object of his belief—it doesn't tell you anything about the world.

Side quest: One popular way of thinking about mental representations is in terms of a mental language called **Mentalese**. This is the **Language of Thought Hypothesis**, which says that thinking happens by means of language-like symbols in the mind. So when I think to myself, "Fido is a dog," I have a sentence of Mentalese in my mind, whose meaning is *Fido is a dog*. Mentalese isn't a language that you speak or are aware of, however. It's the language of the mind that we're all born with. The natural languages that we learn (English, Spanish, Tagalog, Swahili) are mapped onto Mentalese. So the English word "dog" and the Spanish word "perro" are mentally represented in the Mentalese term meaning *dog*.

There have been a lot of objections to the Language of Thought hypothesis, and we think you can find the motivation for one of them right now. What is the difference between how sentences in a natural language acquire their meaning and how sentences in Mentalese acquire their meaning?

(Hint: the big question is, where do thoughts get *their* meanings from? What makes a sentence of Mentalese meaningful?)

"Okay, so we have all this information about disembodiment and minds, but how is all this related to MIND and MATTER?" We're glad you asked. *Both MIND and MATTER assume disembodiment!* Here's how.

3.4 MIND and MATTER—not so different after all

This final section presents a series of arguments to show that MIND and MATTER both assume that the mind is disembodied. While you *could* just take our word for it, we think you should work through the arguments—we might have missed something and you could send us an angry email. Or you might be on the fence and need to be convinced. Either way, it's good practice to work through philosophical arguments carefully.

Here's the plan. We have to show two things: that MIND assumes disembodiment and that MATTER assumes disembodiment. The strategy we're going to follow is to show for each case that *if* MIND (or MATTER) is true, then disembodiment is also true. This shows that disembodiment is a **necessary condition** for MIND as well as MATTER. In other words: if MIND (or MATTER) is true, then disembodiment is true.

To do this, we use something called a **conditional argument**. We assume that MIND (or MATTER) is true. With that assumption in play, we show that disembodiment is also true *because* MIND (or MATTER) is true. We do *that* by taking ideas in MIND (or MATTER) and showing that disembodiment is "hidden" in those ideas.

> **Otto's workbook**: Draw a picture of how a conditional argument works. How can you pictorially represent the assumption that MIND (or MATTER) is true? How can you illustrate that disembodiment is "hidden" in MIND (or MATTER)?

3.4.1 MIND assumes disembodied: the longer explanation

MIND says that the mind "rules over" the body. Remember the example about fitness in the introduction? The idea there was that you can shape your body however you want *as long as you put your mind to it.* Tired? Push through it. Want a slice of cake? Exert your willpower to decline. Whatever your bodily state, your mind can overcome it. If the mind can override the body's desires, then the mind isn't pushed around by the body. Your desires may be influenced by your bodily state, but ultimately, the mind has the final say, which means it works separately from the body. In other words, to even ask "Can the mind 'rule over' the body," is to assume something about the nature of the mind. The assumption is that the mind is a thing we can conceive of as (at least conceptually) separable from the body, with its own kind of abilities to make changes in the world.

The "at least conceptually" in that previous sentence is important. It doesn't mean that minds actually exist separate from the brain. It means that we can formulate theories about the mind and describe its activities separately from what's going on in the brain. In other words, we can treat the mind and its activities as conceptually distinct from the brain.

3.4.2 MIND assumes disembodied: the shorter explanation

Here's another way to see how MIND assumes that disembodiment is true. Go back to our "MIND is true" cases: identity theory and functionalism. For both of these, we have to already understand the mind as working independently of the body. Just stating the position of identity theory requires that mind and body be conceived as separate; identity theory assumes that there are two things to identify as identical in the first place. Functionalism says that the material doesn't matter for understanding how the mind works. In both cases, we don't care about what the body is doing to understand the mind.

3.4.3 MATTER assumes disembodied: the longer explanation

You'll notice that the next part of the argument mirrors the first half pretty closely—just something to keep in mind.

MATTER says that the body "rules over" the mind. And again, let's go back to our examples. When you're hungry, you can be a jerk. The same goes if you haven't had enough sleep or if you suffer from chronic pain. If MATTER is true, then it's your body governing your states of mind. You can't help but behave as you do because your body is in the state it's in.

But notice how we're setting up the dichotomy: it's your mind that is controlled by your body. You believe, want, and feel according to the state of your body. In order to make this claim, the body has to already be thought of as an entity or causal force that's separable from the mind. Here's an analogy: a weightlifter moves some weight by applying force to it. The weight goes in whatever direction the weightlifter pushes (or pulls) it. But the weights are separate from the weightlifter. In fact, the idea of a weightlifter moving weights doesn't make sense without thinking of them as separate things. The same thing goes for MATTER and MIND: to say that our bodily states control our mental states—for example, that I'm irritable because I'm hungry—is to already imagine bodily states and mental states as separate entities. We're thinking of them as distinct things from the very start—and that's exactly what disembodiment says.[13]

The more you know: One of the challenges for embodied theories, as we'll see in Chapter 8, is thinking about mind and body in a way that doesn't leave them in a kind of tug of war. Our argument in the above two paragraphs imagines the body as a causal driver of the mind: the body or brain does whatever it does and we have thoughts and feelings as a result. A question you should keep in the back of your minds is: if that's not how mind and body are related, then how *are* they related?

3.4.4 MATTER assumes disembodiment: the shorter explanation

Go back to our MATTER cases: identity theory (MATTER and MIND are true) and eliminativism (MATTER is true and MIND is false). In both cases, the body is thought of as distinct from the mind. The argument for identity theory is the same as the one in §3.4.2. In the case of eliminativism, the mind doesn't exist as a thing in the world: it's brains all the way down. In both cases, mental states are conceptualized as entities distinct from bodily states, and that distinctness is exactly the hidden assumption of disembodiment we set out to expose.

> **Otto's workbook**: We've done a lot of arguing in a very short space. It can be useful to restate arguments in your own words. So spend a few minutes convincing yourself that (a) mind-over-matter assumes that minds are disembodied and (b) matter-over-mind assumes that minds are disembodied. Some folks find it helpful to write out the ideas in bullet points; others find writing a few paragraphs useful for solidifying ideas.

3.5 Rejecting disembodiment

So what have we seen so far?

We began with a hunch that mind-over-matter could be true, and matter-over-mind could be true. We explored the space of possibilities and found problems with every option. We argued that all the positions we considered suppose that the mind is disembodied. Now it's time for us to ask, "Do we have any good reasons to reject the disembodiment of the mind?"

As you might suspect from a book about embodied cognition, we have good reasons to reject disembodiment. We'll consider four of them.

3.5.1 Conflict aversion

Each philosophical position about the nature of mind that we have considered assumes that minds are disembodied. If we reject the claim of disembodiment, then we can't adopt those views or inherit their problems. So one reason to reject disembodiment is that it lets us avoid a bunch of problems associated with it.

While we're as conflict-averse as the next philosopher, we should note that the disembodiment enthusiast can run the very same argument if it turns out that there are problems with thinking of the mind as embodied. And as we'll see in Chapters 7 and 9, philosophers *have* given that argument.

3.5.2 Double sensation

There's another reason to reject disembodiment: we experience ourselves as embodied. These insights come from a field in philosophy called **phenomenology**. One key insight from phenomenology is that we should focus on our experience of the world and try to bring in as few assumptions about mind and world as possible. We take our experience—every bit of it— seriously, as it presents itself.

The more you know: Phenomenology is an *enormous* area in philosophy and there are disagreements all over the place (as you'd expect from philosophers). **Edmund Husserl** is generally credited as the founding figure. His approach advocated "bracketing" questions about the existence of the world and focusing on our experience of the world. The goal of the bracketing is to give up a particular inclination in how we see the world: namely, as something that is "out there." One insight that perhaps all phenomenologists could agree on is that the division between mind on the one hand and the world on the other is a mistake. What does this mean? Read Dan Zahavi's book *Phenomenology: The Basics* (also from Routledge!) to find out.

Ask yourself this question: which is further away from you, your hands or your feet? This is kind of a puzzling question when you think about it. First, where are we measuring from: our heart? Our brain? Our belly-button? For each of these possibilities, there's a definite answer: our hands are closer to our hearts than our feet are. But it's a weird question in another way: even though there are measurable facts about us, we typically experience ourselves as a whole existing in space. When you think about something as close by (or not), you usually think about it as near or far from *you*, not near or far from your hand.[14]

Here's another one. Press the cover of this book with your right index finger. You're sensing the book's cover: it's smooth and perhaps a little cool. Now press your right index finger against your left thumb. Your thumb feels fleshy and warm. Finally, press your left thumb against your right index finger. Your index finger probably feels fleshy and warm too.

But notice this: when you touched the book, it was you touching an object. The object wasn't feeling you (at least not in any typical sense). But when you touched your index finger to your thumb, you were feeling a part of your body: in the first case, the index finger felt the thumb, and in the second, the thumb felt the index finger. In both of these cases, you are both the experiencing subject and the object experienced. You are both subject and object: the thing feeling as well as the thing felt.

This phenomenon, called **double-sensation**, highlights that the body is both a subject and an object. The body is a subject because it is something that feels; that's what it means to be a subject. The body is an object because it is something that is felt; that's what it means to be an object. This matters because it points out that we aren't disembodied. If we were, we wouldn't have the double-sensation. We would experience our bodies only as objects and never as subjects. If we were disembodied and the mind functioned independently of the body, then the body would be an object to the mind. The body would never be a subject.

Side quest: Phenomenologists have been strongly influenced by a movement in psychology called **Gestalt psychology**. The slogan for Gestalt psychology is that the whole is greater than the sum of its parts. This means that the beliefs and actions of the whole person aren't reducible to the mind's parts. Read about the "principles of grouping" in *Wikipedia* and also look up "holistic facial processing" (which is about how we perceive faces). How does perceiving faces reflect the core Gestalt principles?

3.5.3 Concept of mind

Another set of reasons for rejecting disembodiment comes from a philosophical movement in the mid-20th century called **ordinary language philosophy**. This school of thought argues that paying close attention to our language will show that philosophical problems are often the results of the misuse of language. It also holds that attending to how we talk can reveal new philosophical insights.

The first philosopher we'll consider is **Gilbert Ryle**. In his book *The Concept of Mind*, Ryle offers the following thought experiment. Imagine someone comes to your home and asks for a tour. You show them the kitchen, the bathroom, the bedroom, and the living room. They say "thank you very much for showing me the kitchen, the bathroom, and so on. But I would like to see your *home*." Your guest has made a **category mistake**. They believe that your domicile is something more than the rooms that make it up. But of course, there's nothing more to where you live than the rooms that make up your home. (We mean this in a literal sense, not in a "home is where the heart is" sense.)

Similarly, when people ask about minds, thoughts, beliefs, intentions, and so on, *as separate from behaviors*, they make a category mistake. An intention isn't distinct from the behaviors manifesting that intention. Ryle encourages us to think of talking about the mind using adverbs instead of nouns. To be an organism with a mind isn't to possess a certain thing. Instead, it's to behave in certain ways.

The more you know: A category mistake is another philosophical tool that's really powerful. It says that asking about a certain kind of thing in a certain way is a mistake. So we'll either get no answers or the wrong ones. For example, if someone asks, "How heavy is the color purple?" they're making a category mistake: purple isn't the kind of thing that has weight. So, according to Ryle, when someone asks, "How is the mind related to the body?" they're making a category mistake: minds aren't *things* at all but rather ways of talking about human behavior.

For example, imagine a circus performer who appears to trip and fall, but whose fall is actually a skilled, comic performance. Now compare that with one of the authors of this book, who continually trips and falls because he's a klutz. (We'll call this person "Charlie L." No wait, that's too obvious. Let's call him "C. Lassiter.") We can even imagine that the falling behaviors of the performer and the klutz look the same. What's the difference? Ryle would tell us to avoid saying that the performer had an intention, while the klutz did not. Instead, the performer fell *skillfully* or *purposefully*, and the klutz did not. The difference is in *how* they fell—and how they would fall under various conditions—not in whether one had an intention in mind and the other didn't. The klutz couldn't fall the same way twice; he doesn't have the skills for that. However, the circus performer *can* fall the same way twice because of the skills he acquired in learning to fall in a particular way.

Otto's workbook: Come up with an example in which person A and person B perform the same behavior, but A did it on purpose while B did not. Now point to differences in A's personal history and B's personal history to explain how A did it on purpose and B did not.

What does all this mean? Just that our concept of mind is already embedded in our concept of a body. Ideas like "intention" are really just shorthand for describing how someone behaves or would behave.

Our second philosopher is **Peter Strawson**. Like Ryle, Strawson is keen to point out that our concept of mind already has the concept of a body as part of it. In other words, we can't think about minds without thinking about bodies.

So how does Strawson do this? In his essay, "Self, Mind and Body," Strawson points out that if we know what something is, then we have to know how to count it. That is, to say what a kind of thing is, we have to be able to **identify** and **individuate** instances of it. So, for example, we know how to identify and individuate books. A book is an object made up of pages and typically has words written on them. (Ignore ebooks for now.) We also know how to count books: they have a front cover and a back cover and usually form a single whole. For example, the first 10 pages and the last 10 pages of this book are part of the same book.

How do we identify and individuate minds? The disembodiment theorist says that minds are disconnected from bodies. Following that logic, counting bodies isn't a reliable way to count minds. The next time you're in a crowd, look around. Maybe some of those bodies have minds, and maybe some of them don't. Maybe some of them even share a mind. But since minds are disconnected from bodies, we can't say for sure.

The embodiment theorist, on the other hand, says "Count the people–that's how many minds are in the room." There's a simple rule for counting minds: "*one* person, *one* consciousness; *same* person, *same* consciousness" (Strawson 2008, 191). This is because our concept of mind is derived from our concept of a person, and our concept of a person—of a human being—includes the concept of a body.

Strawson concludes, then, that our concept of mind already has as a part the concept of persons and, therefore, of bodies. There is no thinking about the nature of the mind apart from the body.

3.5.4 Symbol grounding problem

The words on this page are just inscriptions—they don't mean anything by themselves. **Paul Grice** described this as **non-natural meaning.** For non-natural meaning, social conventions are needed for an expression to mean anything at all. "Dog" means *dog* because we language-users agree on that. Smoke, on the other hand, means *fire*; just like a fever means that the person has an infection, and sunburn means that someone has had too much exposure to UV rays. These are cases of **natural meaning.**

Our heads are populated by representations (according to disembodiment theorists). How do these representations get the meanings they have? In other words, how does the thought "my coffee is cold" come to mean *my coffee is cold*?

We have two options: the meaning is non-natural or it is natural. Let's consider non-natural meaning first: maybe the meaning of the thought is a kind of non-natural meaning? The *thought* "my coffee is cold" means *my coffee is cold* in the same way that the *sentences* "mi café está frio" and "my coffee is cold" mean *my coffee is cold*. Sorry, but that won't do. Non-natural meaning always has to get its meaning from somewhere else. If the contents of our thoughts are non-naturally meaningful, then they have to get their meaning from somewhere else. But then we have to ask: where do *those* meanings come from? This creates an infinite regress because every time we identify mental meanings as non-natural, we have to investigate whatever it is that gives those non-natural meanings their meanings. We're effectively saying, "A gets its meaning from B. B gets its meaning from C. C gets its meaning from D…" on and on until the heat death of the universe (and even past that). Usually, infinite regresses mean our philosophizing has gone wrong somewhere.[15]

Let's try the other option: Maybe the meaning of our thoughts is a kind of natural meaning? That would mean that the thought "my coffee is cold" means *my coffee is cold*, just like smoke means fire. The problems with this suggestion are best revealed through a back-and-forth between speakers, so we're going to play out the worry here as a dialogue. (Philosophy is often done this way; Plato's work is written like this.) This dialogue isn't going to win the Nobel Prize, but we're hopeful it'll communicate some big ideas in a digestible way. The disembodiment theorist will be represented by "DT" and the embodiment theorist by "ET."

DT: The thought "my coffee is cold" means *my coffee is cold* just like smoke means fire.

ET: No, that can't be right. Smoke means fire to someone. It's people who make the connection between smoke and fire. Who is the person making the connection?

DT: It's me! I'm making the connection!

ET: But who or what is this "me" if it's not the thoughts in your head? You'd have to exist apart from your thoughts to do that. But then we can ask, "how does the smaller you in your head make the connection between the thought and its meaning?" You'd have to posit ever smaller homunculi to explain this.

DT: Okay, never mind. Maybe it's just a **brute fact** of nature that the thoughts mean what they mean. It just is what it is and there's no deeper you can go. You've reached the end of explanation.

ET: That's possible, but we're left with a mystery. Why on earth should the connection between thoughts and meaning be a brute fact? That's like saying "fever means infection" is a brute fact, but it's not—we have some pretty good biological theories about infection causing fevers. So if it's a brute fact, it's one that doesn't have any kind of parallel in nature. It is, as stuffy philosophers sometimes say, **sui generis**—there's nothing else like it; it's its own genus.

It's possible that the mind is its own genus and doesn't share anything in common with anything else (except other minds), but then the mind is a bizarre entity from the perspective of nature.

DT: Okay, no, I've got it this time. Representations are realized in neural tissue—the neural tissue naturally means *my coffee is cold*, and when I think "my coffee is cold," that's me being aware in virtue of the natural meaning of the pattern of neural activity.

ET: So, for the sake of the argument, a pattern of activity in my frontal lobe means *my coffee is cold* just like smoke means fire.

DT: Yep.

ET: So there's a pattern of neural activity that generates a thought with the meaning *my coffee is cold* and I'm aware of the meaning of my thought.

DT: Yep.

ET: Okay, so there's a natural connection between the brain and our conscious thoughts, just like there's a connection between fever and infection?

DT: You got it. I win.

ET: Okay, one quick follow up.

DT: Shoot.

ET: Your solution says that our brains generate our conscious thoughts. How does that happen?

DT: I dunno. Some nerd in a laboratory can figure that out.

ET: Hold on. What you're talking about is the **hard problem of consciousness**. There are lots of questions about the mind that are challenging to solve but we know how to solve them or at least what a satisfactory conclusion looks like. For example, figuring out how the visual system works is incredibly hard, but scientists know what a good explanation will look like—or at least scientists will know what explanations are up for grabs as plausible. Right now, philosophers and scientists have no idea what a satisfactory theory about the neural basis of consciousness even looks like.

DT: Say more.

ET: Okay, so infections cause fevers. The connection is that raising the body's temperature is part of the immune system's response to infection. Scientists have a sense of how all this works and tell a biological story about it all. There might be disagreements over details, but there is agreement over the basics. In contrast, philosophers and scientists don't have an understanding of what would count as a satisfactory explanation for the physical basis of consciousness. In a nutshell this problem is: how do we even begin explaining consciousness in terms of neurons? How does three pounds of stuff the consistency of tapioca pudding generate conscious experience?[16] How would we know when we got the right answer? We have no idea what an adequate answer even looks like! So you're free to go this route, but it leads to pretty hefty problems.

DT: Okay, let me try something else. So our perceptions are caused by stuff in the environment. I see a cow eating grass and I have a mental representation whose content is *cow eating grass*.

ET: Okay, that sounds reasonable.

DT: Now, barring misperception, bad lighting, and things like that, my mental representations of things in the environment correspond with the things in the environment. My dog-thoughts correspond to dogs, and so on.

ET: Keep going, I'm not sure where this is heading.

DT: Compare that with simple artifacts like a gas gauge or a thermostat. When your gas gauge is pointing to "E," that means your tank is empty. When the thermostat reads 65°F, that means it's 65°F in the house. The "E" means what it means because it correlates with the state of your gas tank. The thermostat reading 65°F means what it means because it correlates with the ambient temperature. Another way of putting this is to say that the "E" reading on the gauge carries information about the state of your gas tank.

ET: Cool story, but how is this connected to the contents of our thoughts?

DT: I'm getting there! Calm down.

ET: *rolls eyes* fine.

DT: There is a causal chain between the state of the gas tank and the gauge reading such that the gauge reliably carries information about the state of the gas tank. So the gauge reading "E" *means* that the tank is empty. In a similar way, my mental representation of a cow as a result of seeing a cow reliably carries information about the state of the world. Namely, there's a cow in front of me.

ET: I'm not sure I'm following. Can you say that one more time?

DT: Sure. *Holds up a coffee mug* you see this mug, yeah?

ET: Yep.

DT: Okay, you currently have a perception of the mug. You have a mental representation right now with the content *DT is holding a mug*.

ET: That sounds roughly right.

DT: Your perception is caused by a complicated biological process involving light bouncing off the mug and striking your retina. This in turn does a bunch of stuff, which ends up with you having a mental representation of the mug.

ET: Okay, I'm following...

DT: And just as the "E" on your gas tank means your tank is empty because of a causal chain, your representation of the mug means there is a mug in front of you because of a causal chain holding between the mug I'm holding and your perception of the mug.

ET: Okay! I think I get it! My mug-thoughts are about mugs because my mug-thoughts carry information about mugs. My mug-thoughts carry information about mugs because there is a reliable causal connection between perceptions of mugs and mug-thoughts.

DT: Exactly! This is the **causal-informational theory of mental content**.

ET: That's a long name.

DT: Yeah, whatever. The important thing is that we have a way to address the symbol grounding problem. My mental representations are grounded by means of a causal connection with the world. It's because there is this reliable causal relationship that my thoughts are connected to the world.

ET: Huh, that's pretty interesting…

DT: Right?!?

ET: I have a couple of follow-up questions.

DT: Fire away!

ET: You said "barring misperceptions" but that's a pretty big exception to carve out.

DT: Philosophers have ways of addressing this problem, but this dialogue is getting too long already.[17]

ET: Okay, well in that case, let me think through the issue of environmental conditions. You mentioned bad lighting affecting perception. If it's twilight, I might look at a cow and think it's a horse or sheep.

DT: Yeah that's true, but you'll see that it's a cow in the daylight.

ET: Oh for sure, but why are we taking daylight as the standard? Why is it that I judge the correctness of my representations during the day but not at night?

DT: Duh, it's because there's more light during the day.

ET: True, there is more light. But that doesn't tell us why we should take daytime as the standard.

DT: It's because you can see more clearly in the day! You're less likely to be wrong about what you see.

ET: Ok, so if I have a mental representation of X and it's caused by perceiving an X in broad daylight, then my thought about X is actually about X.

DT: I think so…

ET: Okay. But that begs the question. Why should I take broad daylight to be the standard? And what about perception in nonideal conditions? If I see a cow at twilight and I perceive it to be a goat, then my thought is still about a goat and not a cow. How does it help to say that if it were the middle of the day, I would instead perceive a cow? That counterfactual doesn't tell me what counts as ideal conditions of perception.

DT: What the…. If you can't see clearly, then those conditions aren't ideal! It's as simple as that!

ET: Okay, so perception under ideal conditions fixes the contents of our perceptual thoughts.

DT: YES THIS IS WHAT I AM SAYING TO YOU.

ET: So when I misperceive under ideal conditions, am I not actually misperceiving?

DT: What the f–

ET: Language!

DT: Sorry.

ET: What I mean is that you're saying, "The contents of our thoughts are set by perception under ideal conditions." But we can misperceive under ideal conditions. I might take a quick glance and think I see a goat when it's actually a cow. We misperceive in ideal conditions all the time! Just think of when you see someone walking and you think it's one person but it's actually another.

DT: Oh dude, I hate when that happens. You're like "Hey friend!" but it's someone you've never met. I feel so dumb when that happens.

ET: Same! But it's weird we feel dumb. It happens to everyone, right?

DT: Totally.

ET: But back to misperception: You're misperceiving even when the conditions are ideal. That would mean that your goat perception is caused by cows; or that the perception of your friend is caused by someone who isn't your friend. So it's not the case that our perceptions are always reliable and that they carry information about how the world is. To go back to your gas tank analogy, sometimes the gauge might say "E" but you actually have a full tank.

DT: Okay, soooooo……

ET: So that means that causal-informational theories still have a significant hurdle to overcome. Namely, *how are the contents of our thoughts determined in cases of misperception under ideal conditions*? I don't think you want to say that sometimes you have goat-thoughts because you're perceiving a cow.

DT: No, not really.

ET: So causal-informational theories do well provided we aren't worried about misperception.

DT: I mean....well....

ET: I'm not saying that causal-informational theories *can't* work. I'm just saying that they have to be fairly sophisticated to account for misperception and explain what counts as an ideal condition.

DT: Nuts to this, I'm going home.

ET: Okay cool. Talk at the same time tomorrow?

DT: Yeah. See you then!

3.6 Complicating representations

We mentioned in the Chapter Overview that we would complicate the concept of representations, and now you're in a position to see why. A representational view of the mind has a lot going for it. It's testable and intuitive. The view has some problems, as we saw in §3.5, but that doesn't mean it has to be junked. There are many embodied cognition theorists who retain the concept of representations. We'll discuss one version of this in Chapter 7. Additionally, we'll consider three more possibilities.

First, you might think that representations are needed for some kinds of cognition and not others. Thinking about the past or the future, for example, means thinking about something that isn't physically present. So it might be that some kinds of cognition demand representations and others don't. So you might endorse non-representationalism for perception but not for planning. This connects with a problem we'll first see in §7.3.2.2 and that will reappear in Chapters 10 and 12: representation-hungry problems. Basically, some kinds of cognition require representations. This first way to complicate our notion of representations basically says, "Okay, some kinds of cognition are representation-hungry, so we'll keep representations for those processes."

Second, some philosophers and psychologists use the notion of **action-oriented representation**. For example, Pete Mandik and Bence Nanay propose that some perceptual representations have as their content something like, "Look left" or "the ball is throwable." In this way, representations of the world include something about how you can act in the world and this action-oriented content makes implicit (or explicit) reference to the body.[18]

Third, you might change your understanding of the concept of representation. Catherine Legg, among others, adopts this route. Her ideas are fascinating and nuanced, and unfortunately, we don't have space here to unpack them in detail. The gist is that *habits* are a kind of embodied representation. Habits—having ingrained tendencies to do something, but that can also be changed—aren't only about practical knowledge. In our experience, students have a habit of writing down anything their teacher enumerates on the board. But we can also develop habits about habits (we'll call them "metahabits"): we have habits for picking up and putting down other habits. These metahabits require being able to think about the past and future, and so can count as a kind of embodied representation.

3.6.1 *What's next?*

In this chapter, we looked at ideas of disembodiment and some reasons to reject them. So what happens when we reject disembodiment of the mind? The obvious answer is that we accept that the mind is embodied—that is, that the body shapes our mental life in some way. But we can go even a smidge further. Bodies are *always* in physical and social environments of some kind. You might currently be holding this book in a coffee shop; Charlie is writing this in his office. So it's not a stretch to go from rejecting disembodiment to considering the possibility that both the body and the environment shape our mental life. And that's exactly where we're headed: toward the hypothesis of the extended mind.

Notes

1 Ibn Sina is best known for the "Flying Man Argument" found in his *De Anima*. He asks us to imagine a person floating, such that they are not experiencing any sensory stimulation. He argues that this person would still be aware of his own consciousness. Hence, consciousness doesn't depend on the body. You'll notice that this argument is very similar to the one given above from Descartes.
2 "Modern" philosophy isn't all that modern. It's typically considered as stretching from Francis Bacon's and Descartes' work in the very late 1500s and early 1600s to Kant and his successors in the 1800s. "Contemporary" philosophy is usually thought of as beginning in the late 1800s and early 1900s.
3 More technically, we don't want to depend on a property that can vary from person to person—it's weird to say that you have more possibilities than me because your imagination is more creative than mine. Instead philosophers will talk about conceivability as a guide to possibility. What's conceivable is what is possible. Conceivability is a property that doesn't depend on the vagaries of human imaginations.
4 https://qz.com/982044/descartes-most-famous-idea-was-first-articulated-by-a-woman
5 See Margaret Boden's *Mind as Machine* for a readable and thorough history of cognitive science until the start of the 21st century.
6 Though by most accounts of the start of the Cognitive Revolution, Turing preceded it.
7 As you might imagine, the history of psychology isn't linear or unified. Jerome Bruner, one of the architects of the Cognitive Revolution, bemoaned the information-theoretic turn. The spirit of cognitivism, according to Bruner, was to explore meaning in context and that meaning is the primary cause of human action (Bruner 1990).

8 There are several ways of interpreting Turing's aim in proposing this test. What we have described is a common one, but there are others. See Diane Proudfoot's paper, "Rethinking Turing's Test" for an engaging discussion.
9 This idea—that a function is computable if and only if it is computable by a Turing machine—is known as the Church-Turing thesis. It's a precise definition of what it means to say that a problem in math or logic is solvable.
10 This connects with our discussion of the symbol grounding problem in §3.5.4. There, we noted that it's not obvious how representations in the head come to have the meanings they do. The connection is this: not only do we have a problem with how the representations get their meanings, but we have a problem with figuring out to whom they are meaningful!.
11 From the diminutive Latin term for "man," *homin*. A homunculus is a "little man."
12 One example includes theories for how we come to form accurate beliefs about what other people are thinking, often called the **theory of mind.**
13 One of the big puzzles for Aristotle was self-movement. As a rule, thing B moves because something else—thing A—sets it into motion, and A and B are distinct things. But when I walk across the room to get my coffee, what is moving me? It's weird to say that it's *me* moving *me*–even weirder if you imagine that each of those "me"s refers to a different thing.
14 There are exceptions to this, of course. If you think about action movies, the hero will sometimes be tied up and they'll have to use a foot to reach an object (a key, a knife) that is crucial for freeing themselves. In these cases, our hero focuses on how far the object is from their foot.
15 This is related to the problem of homunculi we introduced in §3.2.1.
16 In conversation, Tony Chemero—one of the leading lights of embodied cognition in the 20th and 21st centuries—once described the brain as "three pounds of Wondergoo."
17 Jerry Fodor, for example, suggests that misrepresenting depends on accurately representing the world, a position he describes as "asymmetric dependence." Check out *Mental Representations: A Reader* for readings in this area of philosophy of mind.
18 Zoe Drayson (2017) offers an excellent review and critique.

4

THE EXTENDED MIND

4.1 Chapter overview

The extended mind is the idea that parts of the cognitive system exist outside the body. Your phone, for example, remembers important numbers and dates for you. It's not as though *anything* outside your body automatically counts as part of the extended cognitive system. There are criteria that something has to satisfy: is it reliably available? Is it trustworthy? Does it do the same kind of work as what's going on inside your head? In what follows, we start to unpack the extended mind concept, compare it with other theories of mind on offer, and respond to some objections to the extended mind.

4.2 Introduction

At first glance, the body shaping the mind seems pretty intuitive. And if you ask most people, they will agree that the mind and the body are connected, at least somehow. We've got plenty of evidence to show that our bodily lives shape our mental lives. (If I (AK) am about to have violent diarrhea, this shapes my interest in the opera I'm watching right now.) We've also got plenty of evidence to show that our mental lives shape our bodily lives (for example, if I don't think the food on the airplane is going to be very good, I walk across the airport and fill my belly beyond the point of feeling full with slightly less bad airport food). But embodiment is more than this.

Saying that the mind is *embodied* shatters our common notion that the mind is separate from the rest of the world. The mind, as Clark and Chalmers (1998, 7) put it, "...ain't (all) in the head...". It's common to

DOI: 10.4324/9781003356622-5

think of the mind as restricted to the skull, or even as identical to the brain.[1] What's behind this tendency? You could, for instance, replace different parts of my body and I would still be me; you wouldn't really be messing with my mind or any of the essential parts of me that make me, *me*. Right?

Otto's Workbook: Starting at your feet, think about having them removed. As this happens take note of what effect this might have (if any) on your mind. Keep working your way up removing different parts of your body. Where, when, and how do you think this would start to have an effect on your mind: your thoughts, cognition, feelings perception, imagination, etc.–if at all? What happens as you get above the neck? Here make sure you start to get really specific. It might help to have images of the anatomy from the neck up—especially diagrams of different parts of the brain. Think about removing parts of the brain one by one.[2]

Once we get above the neck, something strange happens. This is where folks typically stop and say that we're in the realm where thinking happens, where our mind is located. This is similar–but subtly different from a previous point: we've been talking about *mind*-body dualism, but this is *brain*-body dualism. Lots of people make a distinction between the brain and the body.[3] The brain is where all the mental stuff happens, and the body is where all the "mechanical" reactive stuff happens, like a kind of cause-and-effect machine. The brain tells parts of the body to move around, explore the world, and collect data for the brain to process. Then the brain analyzes the data—that is, performs a series of calculations and judgments about that information—and responds with more commands accordingly (Figures 4.1 and 4.2).

This brain-body dualism is a pretty easy one to slip into. It's really common in American pop culture, where you can find memes like these:

Unfortunately, it's not only theoretically flawed,[4] it's also anatomically inaccurate. It's an anatomical fact that: "*...the brain ain't all in the head...*"

The human brain is made up of *lots* of neurons, roughly 86–100 billion. But *so is the rest of the body*. There are over 15 billion neurons in the peripheral nervous system alone and they run throughout the whole body. If you Google images of the peripheral nervous system, you'll see that they're pretty cool (Figure 4.3). Take this example:*

So, even if we feel there's something special about the brain (i.e., that the brain is where thought happens), given this 15 billion+ anatomical fact:

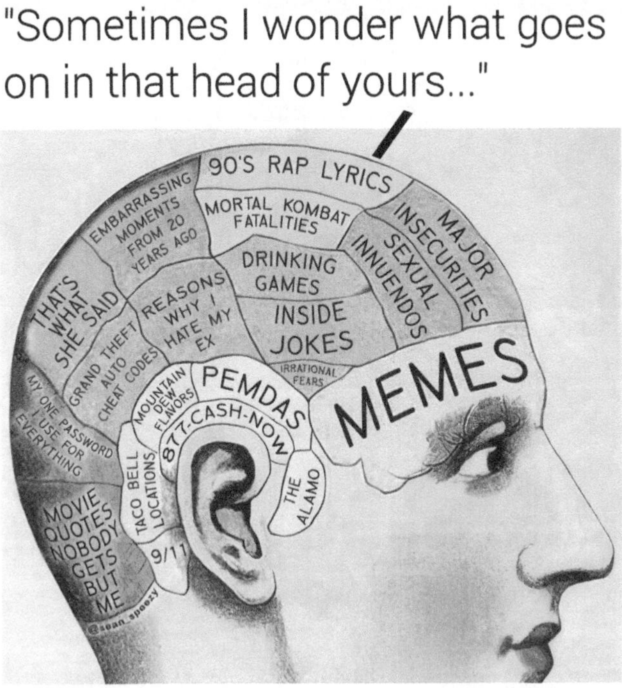

FIGURE 4.1

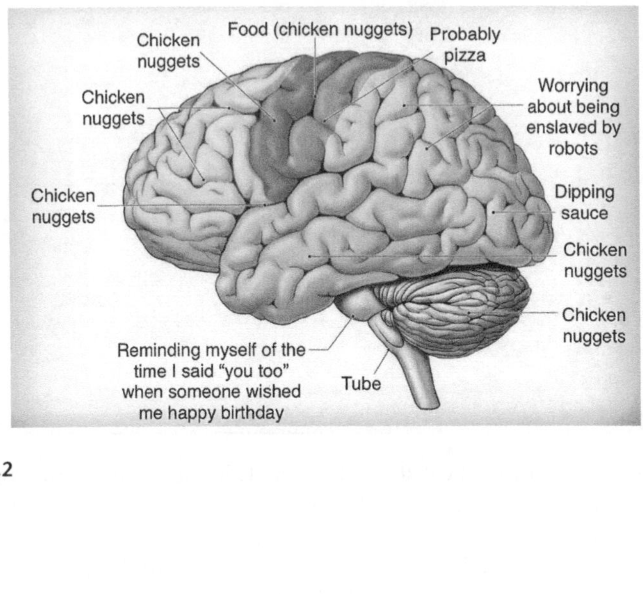

FIGURE 4.2

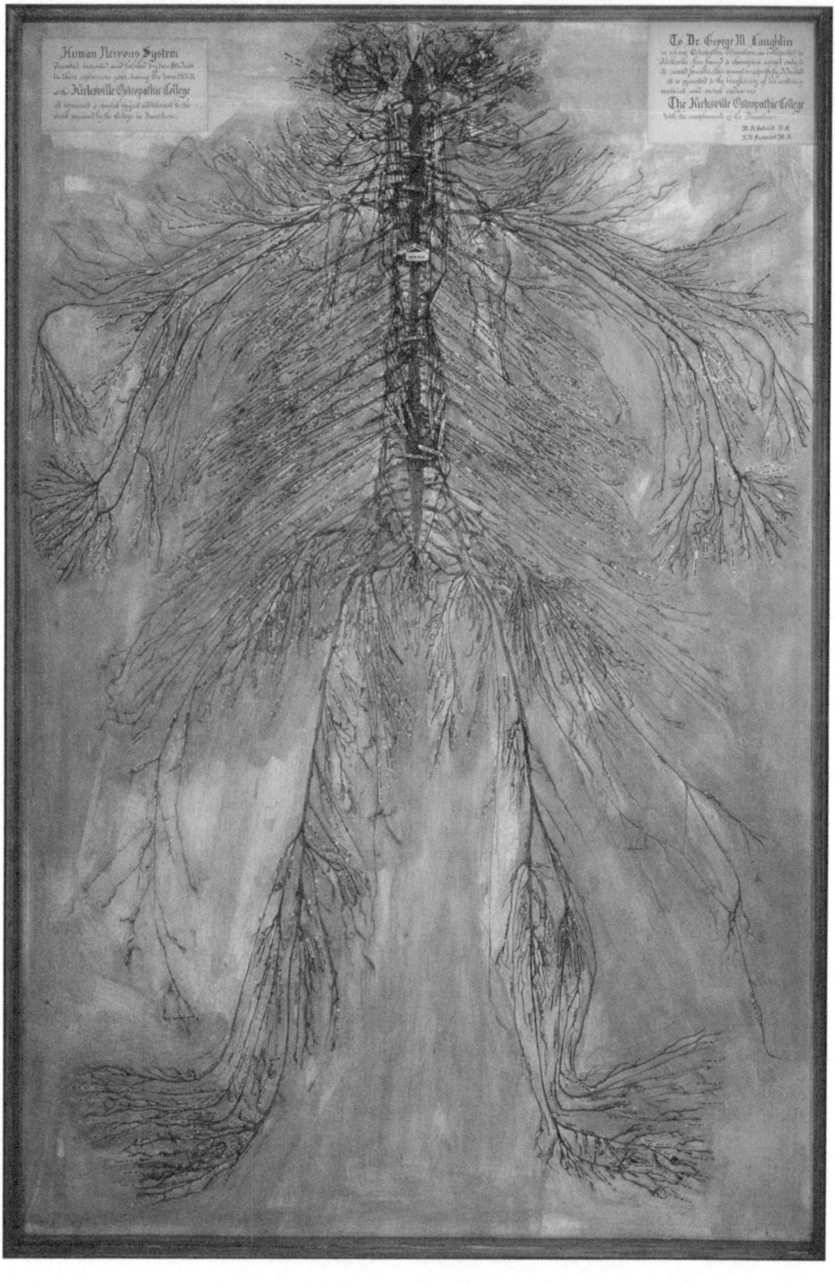

FIGURE 4.3 A pair of medical students spent 1,500 hours dissecting this in-tact nervous system in 1925. (Image credit: Museum of Osteopathic Medicine" (source: Spektor, B. (2018, February 1). *Here's What You'd Look Like As Just a Nervous System*. Live Science). https://www.livescience.com/61599-dissected-nervous-system-photo.html

even if you believe thinking happens in the brain, thought isn't just all in the head—because *the brain ain't all in the head.* Stated differently: the brain is located *throughout* the body[5], so it's inaccurate to think of it as existing entirely within your skull.

This makes things a bit messier and that uncomfortable aporia thing may start to come back. We're so used to thinking of the brain inside the skull that we can have a hard time imagining it as distributed through the body. But don't give up just yet! Understanding the mind as embodied can help us out by taking the mind out of the skull and into the body and the world.

4.3 Embodiment: extending our notion of the mind

If we crack open the notion of embodiment, there's an important concept at its core: the boundary between mind and world is permeable. The mind is *extended.*

Let's start with a simple question:

Where does the mind end, and the rest of the world begin?

The answers to this question are deeply varied and fascinating. Many people (not just nerds like us) have spent their lives asking it. For many of us, the answer starts out the same:

Thought ain't just all in the head...[6]

But where things go from here is wide open. As we'll see in upcoming chapters, this makes things messy and complex. Here's just one way things get tricky:

i The nature of mind: where exactly the mind ends and the rest of the world begins;
ii Consequences of embodiment: what this implies about our existence and everything else in the world (e.g., how we understand perception, experience, consciousness, and lots of other heavy stuff).

But we're getting ahead of ourselves. Let's start with the idea at the heart of all these views: the **Extended Mind Hypothesis.**[7]

What follows is a brief summary of the theory of the Extended Mind (hereafter abbreviated EM). Since the inception of this view (famously articulated by Clark and Chalmers in their 1998 paper), EM has exploded into a rich and exciting school of thought, one that helps us make sense of the world in incredible ways.[8] While there are many ways to develop the core ideas of EM—and we'll be talking about many of them soon—they all center around a common theme, though they differ in the aspects they explore or emphasize.[9] That common theme is: the mind includes the body and world; that is, the body and the world are *part of* the mind.

You can think of the following summary of EM as a kind of "jazz standard," from which there've been countless variations, some we love, some we love less. *Autumn Leaves* performed by Cannonball Adderly sounds very different from Sarah Vaughan's, or Eric Clapton's versions, but they all have the same standard or "core stuff" that makes them (roughly) the same idea.[10] So here's our attempt at the "purest" version of it. We hope you "dig our chops"...

4.4 Extended mind proper

Here's a task for you: Take a note of the day of the week and the date. Figure out the day of the week (not the date!) for the date five days before today's date; do it as quickly as you can.

How did you do it? More importantly, what sorts of things did you do with your body while you did this? If someone were to watch you doing this, how would they *describe your behavior*?

You might have tilted your head up and looked away, turned your body, crossed your legs, moved your head down to block out distractions, or maybe even used something to help you count and keep your place. This short list suggests that our bodies are heavily involved in our thinking. But there's one specific sort of behavior we can focus on. For most of us, there's an easy way to figure this out that you may have done: using your fingers to count and/or "hold" places.[11] Instead of having to keep the dates and days "in mind," you use your fingers to keep track of some of that information.

Side quest: Run the task above by a few other people, five folks would be great. When they're thinking through the problem, note their behaviors. What do they do with their bodies? Do they use their fingers or something else to count? Do they move around? What kinds of things can you observe them doing as they're trying to come up with the answer? Note what patterns emerge between the five people. Why do you think there were similarities or differences?

We do this all the time, using our fingers and hands to count. Sure, you do it when you're growing up and learning to count, but we do it even now, like when you're enumerating items in a grocery list or remembering a set of tasks you promised someone you'd complete. If you don't do this, then your calculations aren't as accurate, your thinking is modified, slowed, or hampered.[12] But what exactly are we doing when we use our fingers? Given the way we use (or rely on) our bodies in the calculation, it stands to reason that this is at least *part* of thought. Why? Because it's doing some of the thinking for us; our fingers are reminders of information we need in order to solve a task.

Central to this is understanding the *way(s)* in which the world is part of the mind, and, in virtue of this, how the process of thinking ("cognition") *extends out* into the world, through our bodies, and into the environment.

Recall what we said about working memory in the previous chapter, à la George Miller. Our working memory is limited; we can only remember so much information before things start to slip. But, thanks to my fingers, I don't have to hold so much information "in my head." I can *enhance* or *scaffold* my memory. According to EM, this is no surprise at all, because, given that I am *reliably coupled*[13] to my hands, they are part of my (outside) memory. My memory is embodied.

Here's another example. When you're listing things out, you might stick out a finger with each item. "I'm going to the store and picking up [sticks out thumb] apples, [sticks out index finger] flour, and [sticks out middle finger] milk." When you get to the store and forget one of the items, you may go through the routine again. "Shoot, I got the milk [sticks out thumb] and the apples [sticks out index finger]. What am I forgetting [wiggles middle finger]?" You're using your hands as part of the remembering process.

Looking past our hands, beyond our bodies, we can also see our thoughts and memories extend beyond the skull. Before the era of cell phones and the Internet, people used to remember a lot of different phone numbers. Today, however, chances are you have maybe a handful that you remember "*in your head*." But if I ask you if you *know* someone's number in your contact list, you'll likely say yes. Why? Because you can quickly, easily, and *reliably* recall this information via your cell phone. Before cell phones, people used to have little notebooks where they wrote this kind of information down and knew exactly where to look for different numbers and kinds of information—some people dog-eared the pages or had a system for indexing them.

According to EM, whatever thing, and/or system, one uses, so long as it allows you to be *reliably coupled* to it—for example, you can reliably access this information—*constitutes* part of your thinking. This is one of the ways that the mind extends out into the world.

> **Otto's Workbook**: What are some other ways that we use our bodies, or things in the world, as a kind of outside memory?
>
> (Think about things that "jog" your memory)

Still not convinced? In a now-classic example, Clark and Chalmers ask us to consider what, if anything, is the *real* difference between what the following people do: (cf. Clark and Chalmers, section 4, "From Cognition to Mind")

- **Otto**, who suffers from Alzheimer's disease, writes down things he learns in a notebook. When he needs that information, he looks it up. He wants to go to the Museum of Modern Art, so he consults his notebook, which says it's on 53rd Street between 5th and 6th Avenues, and then walks to the museum.
- **Inga** also wants to go to the museum. "She thinks for a moment and recalls that the museum is on 53rd Street, so she walks to 53rd Street and goes into the museum..."

Both Otto and Inga want to go to the museum, effectively recall the information, and go there; they both know where the museum is. What's the difference?

You might say that the only real difference is that "...for Otto, his notebook plays the role usually played by a biological memory." So how much of a difference does that make?

For EM, there's virtually no difference:

> For in relevant respects the cases are entirely analogous: the notebook plays for Otto the same role that memory plays for Inga. The information in the notebook functions just like the information constituting an ordinary non-occurrent belief; it just happens that this information lies beyond the skin...

There's no difference because Otto's access to the information is just like Inga's access to the information: it's fast, reliable, and trusted. The only difference is where the information is located. While we don't all use Otto's notebook, most of us certainly have some version of Otto's notebook with us at all times: our smartphones.[14]

In fact, we can make the argument explicit:

Premise 1: If the case of Otto is like the case of Inga, then the mind extends beyond the skull.
Premise 2: The case of Otto is just like the case of Inga.
Conclusion: The mind extends beyond the skull. [Premise 1, premise 2, modus ponens]

Premise 1 is another way of stating the main idea of EM. Evidence for premise 2 was mentioned in the previous paragraph: Otto's access to the information is as readily available and trusted as Inga's access.

These days, many things once realized by biological memory are offloaded or extended through our external memory (i.e., our devices). I no longer remember (in my head) how to get to most places; I use Google Maps. I have always been horrible at remembering what time I have to do things (like when my next meeting is), but thanks to my calendar app, I know where I should be, and when.[15]

4.5 The odd coupling: parity + agent-centric reliability

When we say that thought doesn't just happen in the head and that things like fingers, notebooks, and phones are part of cognition, it *does not* mean that fingers and notebooks are thinking things. This is important to stress because some philosophers have taken cheap shots at EM by treating it like a version of **panpsychism**, a view in philosophy of mind that says everything (i.e., the "pan" part of "panpsychism") has conscious experiences (i.e., the "psychism" part of "panpsychism").[16] For EM, the body and world are part of cognition, but that doesn't mean that inanimate objects think all on their own, like some Pixar movie. Moreover, not just *any* old object or system we engage with is necessarily part of our thought. What matters for EM is *reliable coupling* and *parity*.

What does it mean to be reliably coupled? Clark and Chalmers give this example:

> If the resources of my calculator or my Filofax[17] are always there when I need them, then they are coupled with me as reliably as we need. In effect, they are part of the basic package of cognitive resources that I bring to bear on the everyday world. These systems cannot be impugned simply on the basis of the danger of discrete damage, loss, or malfunction, or because of any occasional decoupling: the biological brain is in similar danger, and occasionally loses capacities temporarily in episodes of sleep, intoxication, and emotion. If the relevant capacities are generally there when they are required, this is coupling enough...
>
> *(Clark and Chalmers p.11)*

Let's revisit functionalism from §2.2.3: mental states are what they are because of their inputs and outputs. But this time, let's think about functionalism with reliable coupling in mind. Functionalism helped us think more broadly about what can count as cognitive: so long as something is functionally equivalent, it doesn't matter what it's made out of (neurons, silicon, paper, etc.), it's part of cognition. But the trouble with functionalism was that it was *too* permissive; almost anything could be a cognitive state (like our China example from Chapter 2). Fortunately, EM doesn't focus only on inputs and outputs but also on how the underlying parts relate to each other. Under EM, for something to be considered part of cognition, it not only needs to realize the relevant function(s) but must also be *reliably coupled* to an (embodied) *agent*. The goal of EM is to make functionalism just permissive enough to recognize something that's patently obvious: we use the world to think *all of the time!*

Here are Clark and Chalmers again:

> If, as we confront some task, a part of the world functions as a process which, were it done in the head, we would have no hesitation in recognizing as part of the cognitive process, then that part of the world is (so we claim) part of the cognitive process. Cognitive processes ain't (all) in the head!
>
> *(Clark and Chalmers 1998, 8)*

While this sounds very functionalist, and indeed it is, EM avoids functionalism's permissiveness problem by adding an extra requirement for something to count as part of cognition: *reliable coupling*. It's not simply that Otto's notebook contains the right information and memories, but that Otto is *reliably coupled* to his notebook in such a way that he can repeatedly and reliably recall the information. That is, Otto's notebook is part of *his* thought(s) because he's reliably coupled to it *and* the notebook "...functions as part of a process which, were it done in the head, we would have no hesitation in recognizing [it] as part of the cognitive process" (Clark and Chalmers 1998). This combination of reliable coupling plus functional equivalence later came to be known as the **parity principle.**[18]

Here's an example of parity without reliable coupling:

Suppose Otto was a bit more like me (AK) and had *all kinds* of notebooks filled with notes, facts, ideas, and important information. These notebooks are unfortunately strewn about my office, some are even tucked away in boxes or stuck inside of other notebooks. Since all of these notebooks can fulfill the function of my extended memory (i.e., there's information that lives there, instead of in my head), does that mean I've got a super big memory? Absolutely not. In fact, the opposite is the case. Why? Because I have no really good idea where any piece of information is stored and in which notebook. If I remember that there's an important piece of information on "human-technology relations" in one of my notebooks, it's useless to me. I have no idea which notebook, where the notebook is, or where in that notebook the information is. I have no *reliable* means of accessing this information. This is because, unlike Otto, I'm not *reliably coupled* to any of these notebooks. I'm not coupled in any consistent or reliable way to these items, so they can't serve to extend my memory.

Think about this the next time you're taking notes in the margins, shelving away a notebook, or putting documents into random folders in your laptop. Ask yourself, can you reliably recall what sorts of notes are in there, where they are specifically, and, more importantly, how they fit within your own thinking? I used to fool myself into thinking I could answer in the affirmative and that I had a pretty fancy system of symbols and notation that I thought would be good. Unfortunately, I didn't see the massive limitation: restricting things to the book itself isn't conducive to my writing or thinking. I've got to remember "Oh, I wrote something about that in my copy of Husserl's *Ideas II*," then open up the book and try to find it, without getting distracted by all the important notes, asides and other "brilliant ideas" that came to my mind when I was reading it in grad school.

So what's the solution here? Clearly, it's important to take notes and write things down. Well, there's a whole school of thought that maintains *any* kind of note you take is pretty much useless unless it reliably and systematically fits into a substantive web of your own thoughts. Notes need to be part of a larger system or serve a function within your thinking. As the author of *How to Take Smart Notes* states:

> ...underlining sentences or writing comments in the margins are also just fleeting notes and do nothing to elaborate on a text. They will very soon become completely useless—unless you do something with them.

The Smart Notes technique(s) and the "Zettlekasten" system on which it was based on are quite popular in many circles, and the techniques, systems, and apps that support this way of thinking and writing are ubiquitous these days. The tools and techniques even have a very catchy EM-friendly name; most call it "building a second brain!"

This agent-centric nature of EM helps keep things grounded; it's the agent's mind that extends out into the world.[19] It's not that things around you can think on their own; nor is it the case that thinking ever happens outside of a context. The big insight of EM is that the world (including our bodies) is part of the mind.

4.6 OK. So what's the big deal?

Otto's Workbook: Now that you know about the core of EM, how much better or worse is it than the previous views? What problems might it solve? What problems might this bring up? Why?

In Chapter 2, we briefly chatted about four views in mainstream philosophy of mind: identity theory, eliminativism, functionalism, and instrumentalism.[20] In Chapter 3, we saw that disembodied views have a number of problems that might be avoided by switching to an embodied view of mind. But as we'll see, no theory in philosophy of mind is free from problems. So maybe there's something to bringing together some mainstream positions and the extended mind. This section is both an exercise in imagining the space of possibilities and checking to see if there are any fundamental tensions between the extended mind and the views mentioned in Chapter 2.

So if EM is true, then what does it mean for the views we talked about in Chapter 2? Does it fit with any of the tried-and-true theories about the mind we saw? Compared to most theories of mind, EM reframes a *lot*, making some views seem patently absurd, while also "playing nicely" (i.e., being compatible with) other theories. With EM, it's hard to draw clear boundaries between what is and isn't the mind. Unlike most ways of thinking about ourselves, there's no sharp distinction between the body, the mind, and the outside world, which puts us in a great position to find new takes on old positions.

4.6.1 EM and identity theory

Identity theory, recall, says that mental states are identical to physical states of the brain. We can supplement the "brain" part of the description with mention of the extracranial world: mental states are identical to physical states of the brain and world. Just as we have fMRI data that can tell us what parts of the brain are relevant and which aren't, cognitive scientists can discern which parts of the world are relevant (Otto's notebook) and which aren't (the north-facing window on the fifth floor of the Flatiron Building).

EM is compatible with identity theory, though it generates some worrisome issues about minds, brains, and pieces of the world. For example, suppose some state of your brain, combined with two different tools causes the same behavior. Here's what we mean:

a $\text{Behavior}_1 = \text{Brain State}_1 + \text{Tool}_1$;
b $\text{Behavior}_1 = \text{Brain State}_1 + \text{Tool}_2$;

But these imply:

c $\text{Brain}_1 + \text{Tool}_1 = \text{Brain}_1 + \text{Tool}_2$.

That seems strange, given that Tool_1 and Tool_2 are (by hypothesis) different things!

4.6.2 EM and eliminativism

Irrespective of debates around whether mental states really exist, EM can either remain agnostic or committed to Eliminativism—either way, EM is compatible here.

Whatever concepts we have or use to explain human behavior, the ones associated with psychological states extend beyond the skin and allow for a less theoretically flawed approach to understanding our mental lives. That is, if mental states are eliminated, it does not change the fact that organisms like us extend our "selves" out into the world.

If, as Eliminativism maintains, all of our psychological language gets eliminated by more precise language about the natural world (or newly discovered natural phenomena), we end up in a world where psychological states go the way of pseudosciences like phrenology and phlogiston theory. What EM adds in this case is that, irrespective of how our scientific theories turn out (or whatever our best neuroscience reveals), we'll need to include more than just the body. As such, EM can maintain either an agnostic or compatible position vis-à-vis eliminativism (at least for now). For example, by looking at the mind as extended, the eliminativist now has a new way of looking at what it means to eliminate mental states or, if you like, a whole new set of things to eliminate.

4.6.3 EM and instrumentalism

There's not much conflict between instrumentalism and EM. In many ways, EM can be "agnostic" about metaphysical claims about mental states. You can be an EM proponent *and* an instrumentalist. You would just be using the EM view over others because it allows for more predictive success in the real world. EM can, for example, be an excellent lens for understanding why people who sit on their hands doing calculations solely "in their heads" perform much worse than people who are allowed to use their fingers.

4.6.4 EM and functionalism

There's not much conflict for EM here either. In fact, EM builds on functionalism.

According to functionalism, so long as a system *functions* in the right sorts of way, we can call it "mental," irrespective of what (physical) stuff the system is made up of.[21]

As we've seen with the standard view of EM, it doesn't matter what a system is made up of; so long as we are *reliably coupled* to it—for example, a notebook, a smartphone, or our fingers—it can constitute thought.

What's different for EM is that it can avoid some of the severe pitfalls of classic functionalism. For instance, Ned Block's objection to functionalism (see Chapter 2) can be avoided because with EM, psychological states can't just be realized out of nowhere. The (extended) pieces or functions that a thing realizes (whether it's a notebook or the coordinated behavior of Chinese citizens) *must* be reliably coupled to an agent. For EM, there are conditions on the integration of the parts constituting the system; functionalism doesn't obviously have those.

So, while EM has a "home" here with functionalism, it differs in that reliable coupling is an essential part of the equation, meaning that EM is a kind of "neo-functionalism."

4.7 Objections to EM

As you might imagine, EM faced a lot of objections. Here we'll cover two of the most prominent ones.

4.7.1 Causal-constitution fallacy

This worry was articulated by Fred Adams and Ken Aizawa over a series of papers and a book. The gist is that causal relationships between things aren't constitutive relationships. Causal relationships are of the form "A causes B," like how heat causes water to boil. Constitutive relationships are of the form "A is part of B," like how a leaf is part of a tree or a piece of marble is part of a statue. Adams and Aizawa argue that these are separate kinds of relationships between things.

Here is the argument:

1 If the mind is extended, then at least some causal relationships are constitutive relationships;
2 No causal relationships are constitutive relationships;
3 Therefore, the mind is not extended. [1,2 modus tollens]

The first premise begins with the assumption that the mind is extended, that is, that either first-wave or second-wave extended mind is right. One of the points that Clark, Menary, and Sutton make in various writings is that the multitude of back-and-forth causal relationships between A and B give us reason to treat A and B as constituting another entity, C. In our original example with Otto, the notebook causes changes in behavior, and changes in Otto's behavior cause changes in the notebook. There are back-and-forth causal relationships between Otto and his notebook. Or consider your phone: you make changes to your phone, and your phone makes changes to your behavior by, for example, reminding you of places you need to be. So *if* the mind is extended, then some causal relationships are enough to count as constitutive relationships.

But, Adams and Aizawa continue that causal relationships are not constitutive relationships. For example, the sun's rays cause photosynthesis in the sunflower's leaves, but that doesn't make the sun a part of the sunflower's leaves. Cooking food makes it easier to digest, but that doesn't make the oven a part of my digestive system.

There have been a number of replies to this objection. We'll give you one.[22] The objection is **question-begging.** To say that it "begs the question" means that it presumes the outcome that it's supposed to argue for. In this case, the objection begs the question about the bounds of cognitive systems. How do we determine the bounds of a cognitive system? We can't do it before doing research about some sort of cognitive system—or rather, we could, but those bounds wouldn't be informed by the sciences. They'd be more or less arbitrary. So we have to do it by being informed by the relevant sciences. We do a bit of research and figure out the bounds of a cognitive system. But that means that we figure out the boundaries in the thick of doing research about cognitive systems; we can't say ahead of time that causally connected systems aren't constitutively related to one another. We discover boundaries by doing some science. Andy Clark describes this using the phrase (borrowed from another philosopher, Daniel Dennett) "cognition is what cognition does." In other words, the bounds of the mind are figured out by looking at how minds work, and minds work through scaffolding in the environment.

4.7.2 Conservativism in science

Science tends to be **conservative**—it changes slowly and tries to accommodate new information into existing theories instead of junking them entirely. Here, that means incorporating our discoveries about the body's role in our mental lives into our current theories about the mind. Theories that are well-established and play important roles in the field tend to be among the last theories to get discarded. For example, if you have to choose between keeping some new theory you've just developed and Einstein's theory of relativity, your new theory is going to be shown the door because Einstein's theory is well-confirmed. We revise scientific theories, of course; psychologists no longer think that you can discern personality by feeling someone's skull. We revise well-established theories when the evidence *overwhelmingly* points in another direction.

In the sciences of the mind, one well-established finding is that the machinery of cognition is located in the skull. To take one of *many* examples, consider Phineas Gage. An accident resulted in a railroad spike going through his frontal lobe. After the accident, Gage was a completely different person. The once friendly and reliable worker was now prone to anger and alcoholism. The explanation is that the damage to the frontal lobe caused the change in his personality. The argument, then, looks like this:

1 Our best theories of cognition suggest that the mind is entirely in the skull,
2 If our best theories of cognition suggest that the mind is entirely in the skull, then the mind is not extended,
3 Therefore, the mind is not extended.

Evidence for premise 1 can be found by opening any cognitive neuroscience textbook and flipping to a random page—OK, maybe not *any* page, but that's not too far off.

Side quest: Read up on any of the following scientists and their findings on *Wikipedia* or in *Foundations of Neuroscience* available free online at the Open Textbook Library: Wilder Penfield, Paul Broca, Patricia Goldman-Rakic, Carl Wernicke, Brenda Milner, V.S. Ramachandran, or Adele Diamond. One thing that they all have in common is that they understand mental activity almost exclusively in neural terms.

For premise 2, suppose that our best theories suggest that the mind is located in the skull. We then have very good reason to think that the mind really is located in the skull. (By analogy: our best theories about evolution suggest that genes are the mechanism by which traits are passed from one generation to the next, so we have good reason to think this is right.) If we have good reason to think that the mind is in the skull, then we do not have good reason to think that the mind goes outside the skull.

The reply here is short and sweet: science doesn't provide certainty and theories are overturned all the time. The history of science is littered with discarded theories. So while current theoretical frameworks in neuroscience may not support the idea that the mind is extended, that isn't the end of the story. After all, there was a time before the germ theory of disease was widely endorsed.

4.8 Conclusions

EM is an exciting theory about the mind because it reframes many of our assumptions about what the mind is and where its boundaries lie. The core idea is that resources to which we're reliably coupled and that do the sort of work that is immediately recognized as cognitive count as part of the cognitive system. Next, we'll take a deeper dive into some of the ideas under the hood of EM. So stay tuned as we begin riffing on some of EM's themes.

Notes

1 We introduced this idea, identity theory, in §2.2.1.
2 This is similar to what Descartes did in his famous *Meditations*. He imagines that an "evil demon" is trying to deceive him about the nature of reality. He could manipulate his senses, make Descartes believe things that aren't true (e.g., 1+1=3), and even cause him to doubt the existence of his own body. But the *one thing*, Descartes believes, that the demon *couldn't* fool him about was that fact that he (Descartes) was still thinking. This, Descartes argues, brings us to the nature of his existence and he concludes: "I think, therefore I am," aka "the cogito," For Descartes, the "thinking thing" is purely mental—an immaterial soul. Nowadays, people often use a similar kind of logic, but rather than identifying the "thinking thing" with an immaterial soul, as he did, they identify it with the brain.
3 See Bering (2006) for discussion.
4 Some common problems for substance dualism include the problem of interaction and the problem of other minds. Suggested readings for Chapter 1 will cover these as well as other problems for substance dualism.
5 Take a quick look back at the side quest. Knowing this and seeing images of neurons throughout the body does this change your answers? Why or why not?
6 You might have noticed that we've used this phrase a couple of times. It's a nod to Hilary Putnam's paper "The Meaning of 'Meaning'" where he says, "meaning just ain't in the *head!*"
7 We intentionally start with the Extended Mind to keep things streamlined and provide a natural route to the Embodied Mind. There are other paths to get to embodiment, but we like this one the best.
8 There are some precursors to EM before Clark and Chalmers. Rob Wilson, for instance, discusses "wide computationalism" just a few years before Clark and Chalmers. And before either of them, there was work in **cybernetics** in the 1960s that has a strong EM flavor. And before *that*, we find themes of EM in the philosophical work of Martin Heidegger and Maurice Merleau-Ponty.
9 As we'll see, for example, an EM emphasis on perception brings us to view of enactive perception.
10 Or their version of the same song.
11 Hold up five fingers, say which day was yesterday and put a finger down, say the day before then and put down another finger. Keep doing this until you have no fingers up and you have your answer. Or, alternatively, start with a close fist and put one finger up as you count backwards each day until you're holding up five fingers. Fun fact, one author employs the former method, and the other one uses the latter.
12 An interesting observation is just *how much* we gesture when speaking. We do it automatically! But it's kind of weird, if you think about it. If speech is just producing sounds, then why on earth would we need to flail our arms about? One hypothesis is that gestures represent features of concepts and that movement helps facilitate use of those concepts (see Robert Krauss's paper, "Why do we gesture when we speak?" for an introduction to this idea). That's not the only game in town for explaining gesture and speech however. The takeaway is to recognize that (a) we gesture when we speak, (b) it's weird, and (c) it's an area of study for psychologists.

13 More on this later.
14 Our heavy reliance on and coupling with our smartphones while very convincing for the central argument of EM also makes things more complicated. But this has more to do with the nature of the system itself, and we'll address this in Chapter 12.
15 And, as we'll see in Chapter 12, with the evolution of different technologies and digital products, my mind has changed even more.
16 Arguably, Adams and Aizawa (2010) think of EM as a kind of panpsychism when they write, "Question: Why did the pencil think that 2+2=4? Clark's answer: Because it was coupled to the mathematician" (p. 67).
17 A company that, during the time of this article, made popular electronic organizers and planners.
18 One of the more pedantic authors (AK) cringes at this phrasing because parity speaks more literally to the concept of *functional equivalence* rather than the reliable coupling aspect. It's in the definition of parity for goodness sake!
19 EM's parity principle has still been criticized for being too vague and permissive. Fortunately, Clark has gotten more specific with his "trust and glue" criteria (e.g., constancy, facility, and trust). For more on this, see Clark and Chalmers (1998, esp, p.15–18), Clark 2003, and Clark 2008, for example.
20 In the "no matter, no mind" category, we mentioned two other positions: minds are just subatomic particles (because everything is ultimately composed of subatomic particles) and minds are really just reflections of the dominant culture (i.e., "anthropology is all you need"). We're not discussing these in relation to the extended mind because in both cases they skip over not only minds but also brains and anything to do with individuals, really. Instrumentalism, though it falls into the "no mind, no matter" bucket, nonetheless addresses behavior by individuals.
21 The tagline of functionalism is: "The matter doesn't matter."
22 This is a reply we have developed and defended in Kagan and Lassiter (2013).

PART 2

Refining the theories

5
INTERLUDE

5.1 End of part 1

We first experienced a kind of confusion, or *aporia*, in thinking about mind and body: sometimes it's "mind over matter"; other times it's "matter over mind." There are exceptions to each of these: hustle culture encourages a mind-over-matter attitude, and consuming too many laxatives confirms "matter-over-mind." We tried to make some sense of this by arguing that both ideas—"mind over matter" and "matter over mind"—assume that minds are disembodied: mind is a thing that works independently of the body.

We explored how this idea shows up in sciences and philosophy of mind and saw that an important idea associated with disembodiment is mental representations. Thinking is a matter of storing, manipulating, and retrieving mental representations. These are sometimes thought of in terms of a kind of mental language, but there are other kinds of mental representations that are not language-like, such as pictorial representations. In the same chapter (Chapter 3), we showed some problems that representationalism faces: the symbol grounding problem, the homunculus problem, and the issue of non-derived content. These problems are substantial enough to encourage us to look elsewhere for an understanding of the mind.

Then we discussed the extended mind. This position says that things outside the head can be part of the cognitive system. But not just *any* thing is part of the cognitive system. There are two considerations. First is the

DOI: 10.4324/9781003356622-7

Parity Principle: something outside the head is part of the cognitive system whenever that thing, if it were to do its job inside the head, would be tagged as cognitive. Second is reliable coupling. Not only does the thing have to be functionally similar to what's going on in our noggins, but we have to have *reliable access* to it and a dense back-and-forth between the body and the thing outside it. This view is neo-functionalist. It's functionalist because mental states and parts of the cognitive system are described functionally in terms of what they do. It's "neo" because it allows the cognitive system to loop outside the head, but *with caveats* like the parity principle and reliable coupling.

It might seem our problems are now solved. And as easy as it might be to write a much shorter book and conclude here, we've still got some important work to do.

5.2 Stress testing EM

One of the things that philosophers like to do is stress-test philosophical positions. What we do is take some idea and see if we can break it. What does it mean to "break" it? A common way is to use the idea to generate absurd conclusions. We've seen this already in Chapter 2. Ned Block argued that, on functionalists' own terms, if functionalism is right, then the nation of China could be conscious. But this seems ridiculous! This is what we mean by "stress-testing" and "breaking" a position.

So far, we've set up extended mind as a binary position: something outside the body either is or is not part of the extended cognitive system. In other words, that "something" outside the head is either a part of the cognitive system (i.e., it helps *constitute* the system) or it causally contributes to the operation of the cognitive system. Whenever you have a binary, an easy way to break it is by introducing tons of "iffy" cases–cases where it's hard to say "yes" or "no." We'll see some of these in the next chapter. Here, we want to describe a few ways that philosophers can respond to the introduction of iffy cases.

First, you can double down on the dichotomy. Your iffy cases *really are* either cases of extended mind or not. We may not be able to tell at the moment, but more work will help settle the matter.

Second, you can blow up one end of the dichotomy. This way says that *everything* is a case of one of the binary options. Here, this amounts to saying either "everything is part of the extended mind!" or "nothing is part of the extended mind!" (i.e., the mind is not extended).

Third, you can insert some buckets between the dichotomy. "Extended" or "not extended" aren't your only choices. Maybe there's "partly extended," where it satisfies some conditions (e.g., functional similarity) but not others (e.g., coupling).

Fourth (and finally), you could say "to heck with the dichotomy!" and treat middling cases as points on a spectrum. The end points you treat as **limit cases**: they're like perfect representations of whatever end they're representing—perfect cases of extended cognition, for instance. All other cases are closer or further away from the limit cases.[1]

Stress testing approaches

	What to do with iffy cases	*So things outside the head are…*
i. Optimist	It's either EM or it's not, we just have to do some more digging and figure it out.	Either constitutive *or* causal.
ii. Binary	Either everything is EM or nothing is	Either constitutive *or* causal.
iii. 2+ options	Create "subdivisions" based on certain conditions	Judged based on additional criteria (e.g., "Partly extended," if parity, but no coupling)
iv. Spectrum	Figure out where they lie on the spectrum between two extremes	Placed on a continuum between limit cases

In addition to treating binary cases in this way, we've seen that there are lots of different cognitive capacities: vision, touch, memory, etc. It could be that, for each of these capacities, there's a different way to treat dichotomies. For example, one theory of embodied cognition takes the second strategy for perception: *every* instance of perception is an instance of extended perception. That is: understanding perception requires understanding relationships among the brain, body, and world. This same theory might have nothing to say about memory or language.

When we do this, something weird happens. What begins as a relatively well-defined and straightforward idea gets *really* complicated *really* fast. Maybe visual perception is best understood by ditching one of the dichotomies, but that doesn't mean we have to treat auditory or olfactory perception in the same way. The range of positions and ideas to explore explodes in number, *but that's okay!* This is part of the fun of doing philosophy. We find ourselves in a kind of wonderment about the possibilities for thinking about the mind and its activities.

5.3 So what's coming up next?

Even if you're not sold on EM, we hope you're at least starting to think differently about the relationship between mind and body and can maybe even find some relief for that pesky aporia that keeps flaring up when thinking about these issues.

In the next part of the book, we're going to continue developing variations of the EM theme. All those things we glossed over and said that we'd get to later—we're going to get to them now. While every view has its own set of problems, our aim is to get to a point where we give you enough of a tour of this area to make up your own mind.[2]

We think these are promising views. All theories have their problems, but the problems that come with these are easier to address than those raised by other views. They also seem to support a lot of emerging empirical science, which we'll discuss, and have some incredible implications for the future of technology, which we'll return to at the end, So in this next section, we'll dive into these variations to show where things are going, what views are available, and what problems and strengths each brings. In short, we believe that embodied views of mind point to new ways of thinking about ourselves that are eye-opening and, in their own ways, startling.

In Chapter 6, we'll be more systematic in exploring the middle space between what *constitutes* mental functions and what merely *causally contributes* to them. We just saw that there are different ways of handling borderline cases with a binary. Since we have to finish writing this book sometime before we retire, we'll adopt this last option: the spectrum approach. We prefer this strategy because it leaves room for a richer range of possibilities and imposes the fewest constraints on how to organize them.

In Chapters 7 and 8, we're going to introduce and then criticize one development of embodied cognition, what we're calling *weak* embodied cognition. It's "weak" in the sense that it retains many tools from the representationalist view of mind while still treating the body as an important constituent of cognition. On the causal-constitution spectrum, weak embodied cognition is smack in the middle, perhaps even shuffling towards the causal end. In some cases the body constitutes cognitive activity, but not always.

In Chapters 9 and 10, we'll introduce and criticize another development: *strong* embodied cognition. This view ditches the tools of representation and introduces alternative concepts for understanding the mind. On the causal-constitution spectrum, strong embodied cognition pulls hard towards the constitutive end: the body is involved in every aspect of our cognitive lives.

With all that in place, let's explore the rich varieties of embodied cognition.

Notes

1 If it's helpful, think about limit cases like geometry. With the curve given by $y = 2/x$, as values of x increase, y gets smaller and smaller. As x goes to infinity, the limit of the function is 0: y will keep getting closer to 0 without ever reaching it for any specific finite value of x.

2 Triple pun intended.

6

INTERPRETATIONS OF THE EXTENDED MIND

6.1 Chapter overview

The parity principle is central to EM. If certain functions happen "in the head," we have no problem calling them cognitive. But what's so sacred about their occurring in the head? If a function happens outside the head, why not also call it cognitive? We explore the parity principle in greater detail and use it to expand what counts as part of the cognitive system.

With this in place, we're now ready for some variations on the theme.[1] We then examine approaches that occupy roughly the same "philosophical camp" as EM but differ in emphasis. Just like different musicians playing "Autumn Leaves," there *are* central themes or commitments, but each each version develops the idea in its own direction. They are all still against the idea of the body as a passive recipient of sense data and reject the notion that cognition takes place only in the head (especially in representational form). Instead, they embrace the role of the body, the environment, and the role of action.

6.2 Parity and complementarity

In Chapter 4, you were introduced to Clark and Chalmers's seminal paper "The Extended Mind" in which they introduce the extended mind. The lynchpin of their position is the Parity Principle. The Parity Principle is about functional similarity: external processes are cognitive if they function like internal ones. We also need reliable coupling: something counts as

DOI: 10.4324/9781003356622-8

part of the extended cognitive system if the Parity condition is satisfied and that something outside you is reliably coupled to you.[2]

A common way to apply the extended mind is as a binary: yes/no, 1/0—looking at something as either extended or unextended. But it's not obvious that the mind works like that. (We're going to see in Chapter 9 that the mind/world boundary can get *really* fuzzy.) Think about the following cases. In particular, each concerns wether one thing is part of another *or* one thing merely causes another:

- Some people hold on to an object as a way to remind themselves of a loved one. You might not always be able to find it or get to it: maybe it's a love letter tucked away in a book that you stumble on every few years. Even though it acts as a reminder of your loved one—and a reliably working one at that—you may not be reliably *coupled* to it.
- A common strategy for remembering where your keys are is to place them on hooks by the front door. This obviously eases cognitive burdens and satisfies some notion of reliable coupling, but do the hooks count as part of your mind?
- Maybe you're like us in that there are some days you want to walk into the forest and never look back. Unless you have the right training, we don't recommend it. *But* you can spend some time with the "24/7 wildlife in the forest" stream on YouTube. Is this a case of extended vision? It's not clear that it is, even if you're reliably coupled to the app.
- If you have a smartphone, you're reliably coupled to search engines. But it seems wrong to say that you know everything on the Internet just because you can Google it.

Otto's Workbook: Come up with 2–3 more examples of cognitive activities that are boundary cases of cognitive extension.

One way to respond to these sorts of cases is to think about the extended mind in terms of a *continuum*. Some processes can closer to the cleaerly extended end, and some show up on the other end, the *causal* end.

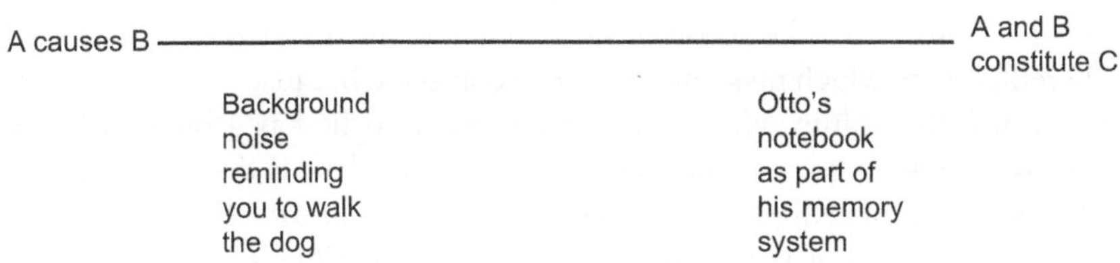

What the continuum tracks is **reliable coupling.** To say that something is reliably coupled to you is to say that you have regular access to it and trust it. But access can be more or less regular; you may trust the object (or person) more or less. For these reasons, reliable coupling isn't all-or-nothing. It's more-or-less. Something is more clearly on the "constitution" end insofar as you are more reliably coupled to it. Something is more clearly on the "cause" end insofar as you are less reliably coupled to it. What this shift in understanding the extended mind does is make space for developing more detailed and sophisticated versions of the theory. We're effectively saying, "you think these examples are decisive objections? They only make us stronger."

There is a principle that we can use to replace the Parity Principle: the **Complementarity Principle.**[3] This principle says that things and processes outside the head count as cognitive if they complement our bodily and mental abilities. While Parity focuses on something outside the head being cognitive if it *works* like something that would be cognitive if it were internal, Complementarity emphasizes something outside the head being cognitive if it meshes with what we can already do.

Let's talk a little more about what we mean by "complementary."[4] When something outside the head "complements" something inside the head, the something outside the head integrates with the standard set of human cognitive abilities.

> **Otto's Workbook**: Offer an argument for why or not binoculars count as cognitive according to the Parity Principle.

The Complementarity Principle offers a new way of conceptualizing what counts as cognitive and why. It's not just that your phone does something *functionally similar* to what happens in your head. Instead, it's that your phone *complements* what you can already do. It *meshes with* your on-board abilities. The external resource and your on-board abilities (e.g., visual perception, memory) create a new kind of thing. The external resource amplifies and, in a sense, generates capacities you didn't have before.

Here's another example of complementarity. My (CL) department chair has a mess of sticky notes covering the desk in his office. Each one has a "to-do" item, and as he accomplishes each item, he discards the sticky note. He remembers which tasks he has yet to complete because they're on sticky notes in front of him. He also doesn't forget that he has a bunch of tasks because the notes are a visual reminder whenever he sits down at his desk. This is a case of complementarity: *the environment and the abilities you already have enable you to accomplish some cognitive task.* In this case, my department chair's visual, motor, and memory abilities (among others) complement his working environment in remembering what tasks need to be finished. He remembers what needs to be done because he has organized the environment in a way that better enables him to do that. It is my department chair and his office that are the cognitive system. In fact, the Complementarity theorist wouldn't emphasize how the sticky notes and his memory are the same. The Complementarity theorist would play up their *differences* to more clearly identify the points of contact: that is, where and how the meshing happens (Sutton 2010).

> **Otto's Workbook**: Describe the case of Otto and his notebook (described in Chapter 4) in terms of *complementarity* instead of *parity*. Specifically, what is it about Otto and the notebook that enables them to dovetail?

Why is this important?

First, it increases the scope of what counts as cognitive. It's not just what's functionally similar but also what complements our bodily capacities that count as cognitive. As a result, physical and social spaces can count as part of the cognitive system.

Here's an example we'll come back to a few times in this chapter. Classrooms are typically organized so that the students sit in desks facing the teacher and the whiteboard.[5] Organizing the space in this way encourages students to stay focused on the teacher at the front. This organization makes it easier for students to attend to the teacher. You tend to look in the direction your body is facing; facing your teacher facilitates looking in their direction and attending to what they have to say.

You might have experienced a failure related to this. Imagine your teacher asked you to sit in a circle and you find yourself sitting with your back to the whiteboard. Suppose your teacher jumps up and begins writing on the board. You have to turn around to see what's happening at the front. You have to exert some energy—and likely strain yourself to turn 180°—in order to see the board. It's now *harder* for you to attend to what the teacher is saying and doing because you have to resist your body's tendency to face forward. The example suggests that positioning the desks to face forward facilitates attending to the teacher. The classroom environment counts as cognitive because it works with our bodily dynamics to support paying attention to the teacher.

> **Otto's Workbook**: When desks are arranged in a circle, what kinds of cognitive activities are they well-suited to support?

Second, complementarity offers a new way of conceptualizing what counts as cognitive and why. It's not just that my phone does something *functionally similar* to what happens in my head. Instead, it's that my phone *complements* my on-board abilities. This might seem like a small shift, but it has big implications. With Clark and Chalmers's functionalist criterion, the question to ask is, "Does this thing work like what's in my head?" (More precisely, "If this thing were to do its job in my head instead of outside it, would it count as cognitive?"[6]) The Complementarity Principle asks, "How does this thing mesh with what I can already do?" The Complementarity Principle requires consideration of our bodies, our behaviors, our environments, and the relationships among all those things. It's a different way of thinking about the world. When we imagine reliable coupling along the lines from Chapter 4, we're not only coupling with specific, token objects like smartphones. We also think about how we cognitively "fit" with the world around us. We'll explore this idea some more in Chapter 9, but there's a kind of mutual fit between us and the world. Our abilities fit with the world we live in, and the world we live in fits with our abilities.[7]

6.3 Getting into the weeds[8]

Our discussions so far point to a few key ideas in understanding the mind, but there are some distinctions we can make. Each one gives us a different flavor of the embodied mind. Let's get into the weeds.

6.3.1 The body

First, the *body* is important. Think about the classroom example we just discussed. Part of the reason why pointing towards the front of the class makes attending to the teacher easier is because of how our senses work. Our peripheral vision doesn't give us the kind of detailed perception of the world that our central vision does. If you're going to discriminate among letters and words on the board, you'll need to use central vision; you'll need to face the whiteboard. Additionally, the construction of your neck and spine matters. The default setting is to face forward. Turning your head requires moving away from the default setting. Putting the teacher at the front of the class works with the natural construction of our neck and spine.

In this short example, we get two ways of thinking about how the body is part of cognition (they're not obvious now, but we hope they will be). First, consider the role of the eyes. The eyes enable you to have access to the information on the board. Here, the body plays a role in cognition, but it doesn't require too much tweaking from the representationalist view we discussed in Chapter 3. You can think about the information on the board by virtue of seeing it, and the role of the eyes is to make that information accessible to you. Eyes are part of the explanation for how we acquire visual information, but the actual information processing still happens entirely in the brain, even if the structures of the eyes and the brain affect how that processing happens. We'll discuss this in greater detail in Chapter 7. We're calling it "weak embodiment."

But now consider the role of the spine. Here, we're going deeper into the body in thinking about its role in cognition. The way your spine is structured plays a role in where your face is pointing and what you are attending to. Your spine might not be a receiver of information, but it plays a role in what you're attending to and what you're thinking about. Your head tends to face forward because that's what requires minimal effort on your part: fewer muscles are needed compared to when you turn your head left or right. The mechanics of the body play a crucial role in our cognitive capacities. You pay attention to your teacher because they're likely an engaging and brilliant professor *and* because of how your spine works. The mechanics of the spine are part of the explanation for why you attend to the board.[9] It's also part of the explanation for why we pay attention to and value some things over others. We will call this "strong embodiment" and will discuss it in further detail in Chapter 9.

The underlying question we'll come back to is: *what is the role of the body in cognition?* We're going to take a deep dive in Chapters 7–10.

6.3.2 The environment

Second is the environment. We've seen how this matters. So much of the built world, from our phones to our classrooms, is organized in order to support our cognitive capacities.

However, there's a distinction here that we've been ignoring. Extended mind advocates say that the environment is *part of* the mind. But do you have to go that far? Can't you say instead that the environment matters, but it's *not* part of the mind? Indeed, you can. The difference here is a **metaphysical** one about the boundaries of the mind. To make sure the environment gets its due in our understanding of cognition, do you need to locate the boundaries of the mind *outside* the body? Or can you keep the boundaries of the mind *inside* the body and argue that the environment *contributes to* the workings of the mind?

Many philosophers and scientists agree that the environment is important for understanding cognition, but they do not go so far as to say that the environment is literally *part* of the mind. This more conservative position is called **embedded cognition.**[10]

Let's introduce an example of embedded cognition. As I (CL) am writing this, I'm sitting at my desk in my office. It's June, and the morning is unusually cool for this time of year—a welcome relief from the unusually high temperatures last week. I have my lukewarm coffee nearby. I'm surrounded by books, journal articles, and scraps of paper with ideas and to-do lists. As I was trying to think of the examples mentioned in this chapter, I would sit back in my chair and look at my bookshelf. Looking at the books helped jog my memory, and I was able to think about examples to make my points.

This is an example of embedded cognition. I'm thinking, and the physical and social context of my thinking is a crucial part of the process. If I weren't in my office, I would have had a harder time coming up with the examples because I didn't have my books to help me think of them. Embedded cognition acknowledges that cognition takes place in an environment and that the environment informs the thinking. For embedded cognition, the environment *scaffolds* the mind but isn't properly part of it.

The more you know: Embedded and extended cognition sound *really* similar: They both emphasize the role of the environment. So what's the difference? It's largely a philosophical one—the extended mind says that stuff outside the head is literally a part of the machinery for thinking. Otto's notebook is literally part of his mind. Embedded cognition says that the environment supports our thinking, but it's not part of the mind. The difference is with the boundaries of the mind: the extended mind supporter says the boundaries of the mind include stuff outside the brain. The embedded mind supporter says that the boundary of the mind is the skull.

"Who cares?" you might be thinking. It turns out that some important things can depend on this distinction. One is how cognitive scientists do their work. If the mind includes things outside the body, then environments immediately become part of what cognitive scientists have to think about in theories of mind. Another is how we think about ourselves. If things outside of us are part of us, then losing that thing is literally losing a part of ourselves. That token from an old friend that reminds you of them? Losing that is losing a memory. A final one is how to think about education. If your calculator is part of your mind, then not being allowed to use one seems punitive and unnecessary—like telling someone to tie their shoes with only one hand. Could you do it? Sure, but it's a lot harder and unnecessary if you have two hands.

6.3.3 The body in action

Lastly, the extended mind encourages us to think about the body in action. When Otto retrieves his notebook, he's moving his hand into his pocket, grasping the notebook, pulling the notebook from his pocket, and opening it. These actions are part of Otto remembering where the museum is. Emphasizing the role of the body is known as **enactive** cognition, or just "enactivism." This view is a serious reorientation from the view of mind introduced in Chapter 3, so let's go through some examples to illustrate.

- Perception of the world requires having an idea (even if not fully describable) of how your sensory impressions change as you move. Perception is not something that happens to us, but rather is something that we *do*.[11] It emphasizes the action or activity of an organism as it navigates the environment and how this implicit bodily knowledge *constitutes* the character of experience. For instance, moving towards an object makes it take up more room in your visual field; moving away from a source of sound makes the sound quieter. These are sometimes called **sensorimotor contingencies**. It's through these sensorimotor contingencies that we experience the sense that we're moving closer to or farther away from things.
- We reorganize problems to make them easier to solve. If you have to divide a pizza into eight equal slices, you won't begin by estimating one-eighth of the pizza. You'll start by cutting the pizza in half, then cutting that in half, and then cutting each of those four sections in half. You've simplified the problem of dividing a pizza into equal slices by doing something to the pizza to make the problem easier to solve. These kinds of actions are called **epistemic actions**.

It's common to think about cognition in terms of what you know: you know *that* water boils at 100° C and *that* wool smells kinda gross when soaked. This is **propositional knowledge**, sometimes called "knowing-that" (notice the presence of "that" in the previous examples). Propositional knowledge is commonly thought of as the key sort of knowing in any kind of cognitive task. This is the kind of knowledge that is encoded in representations, as we discussed in Chapter 3. Enactivists, however, emphasize **practical knowledge**, sometimes called "know-how." Practical knowledge is about *how* to do something. Imagine you want to communicate to someone how to make a peanut butter and jelly sandwich. You have two choices: write down a set of directions going through each step or show them how to do it. Writing down the directions is harder than it seems. For instance, imagine you have "put the knife in the peanut butter" as an instruction—which end is to be put in? "Spread the peanut butter on the bread"—which side? How much of each side? How much peanut butter? Propositional knowledge of making a PB&J isn't as useful as practical knowledge. It's far easier to just show someone how to make a PB&J.

The more you know: In **epistemology**, a persistent question concerns the relationship between propositional and practical knowledge. A longstanding debate asks: is practical knowledge reducible to propositional knowledge (at least in principle)? Some argue that practical knowledge is definable in terms of propositional knowledge: all know-how is really just know-that. Others reject this: know-how isn't definable in terms of know-that. Strong embodiment theorists (like Alva Noë) are inclined to argue that know-that is really just know-how.

6.4 Tuning knobs for theories of embodiment

The features we introduced—bodies, environments, bodies in action—are important for understanding embodied cognition. But these aren't all-or-nothing features: you don't choose one at the expense of others. They are facets of understanding how cognition is embodied, and each one can be more or less important.

It's helpful to think about the different facets as tuning dials with low and high ends.[12] These knobs move you nearer or farther from a disembodied idea of the mind—the sort of mind we encountered in Chapter 3. If you turn up all the dials, you get a conception of mind that is deeply and thoroughly connected with body and world—so much so that it's nearly inconceivable to think about minds along the lines of brains in vats.[13] On the other hand, you can turn down the dials to get a conception of mind that owes a lot to disembodiment and tips its hat toward embodiment.

How do you know if you're dealing with the low end or the high end? The low end will usually use a lot of the ideas we found in Chapter 3. In particular, these sorts of embodiment theorists are fine with talking about mental representations or inferences in perception. For example, Susan Goldin-Meadow researches how gesture affects thought. Even though she argues for the importance of embodiment, she still describes the inner workings of the mind in terms of mental representations.

These notions are conspicuously absent at the high end. You'll find concepts that are more at home in our example with Otto from Chapter 4 and the examples given earlier in this chapter. For instance, we saw that second-wave extended mind is characterized by complementarity: environments and things outside the mind complement (or "fit with") our on-board mental resources. Complementarity-driven extended mind sets the body and enactive dials to mid and the environment to high. So ideas about embodiment at the max-power end will typically make reference to the coupling or connection of mind and world. Strong embodiment (introduced briefly above) sets the "body" knob to "high." Typically, you'll find the "environment" and "body in action" knobs set to medium or high, but it's not required. Behaviorism (mentioned in Chapter 3) sets the "action" and "environment" dials very low while the "body" dial is maxed out.

6.4.1 Theories and their frequencies

We've introduced a few theories about the mind so far. It is helpful to put them all on a common measurement to compare them.

Theory	*Where discussed in the book*	*Body*	*Environment*	*Action*
Disembodiment	Chapter 3	Low	Low	Low
Parity principle extended mind	Chapter 4	Mid	High	Mid
Complementarity extended mind	Chapter 5	High	High	Mid
Weak embodiment	Chapter 7	Mid	Mid	High
Strong embodiment	Chapter 9	High	High	High

We hope this is a helpful way to identify how the different theories are similar and different.

The more you know: Remember in Chapter 2 when we tried out different combinations of MIND and MATTER and truth and falsity? That helped us identify the space of possibilities for MIND and MATTER. We can do the same thing here! We have three categories (body, environment, action) and three options for each category (low, mid, high). That's $3^3 = 27$ combinations. Using this framework, we can give some details about 27 different ideas about the nature of mind. Some of them might not make sense and others might. But the real power in this exercise is seeing all the possibilities for developing a theory of mind. Think that the environment is important but the body and action aren't?[14] Set your dials to "high" for environment and "low" for everything else.

6.5 Conclusion: Signal and noise in thinking about the mind

The metaphor of "signal" and "noise" comes from engineering and information theory. Imagine you're trying to have an intimate conversation with a friend at a rowdy club: that's a lot of noise obscuring the signal. Now imagine you're trying to have that same intimate conversation in your living room or kitchen: that's very little noise obscuring the signal. Lots of noise requires very strong signals to be detected; little noise doesn't require signals to be as strong. A lot of noise with a weak signal can drown out the signal.

So in thinking about the mind, what's signal and what's noise? What's important in thinking about the nature of mind and what isn't? Turns out that the question is *really* hard to answer. Well, "really hard" depending on who you're talking to. What we can do at this point is sketch how we might begin answering the question.

So what are some of the things we've talked about as important? Here's a short list:

1. The brain;
2. The body;
3. The body in action;
4. Objects in our environment;
5. The local physical environment;
6. The social environment;
7. The cultural environment;
8. Humans' evolutionary development;
9. Our subjective experiences;
10. Relationships among items 1–9 in this list.

Now, depending on what vision of embodiment you subscribe to, some of those things can be signal, and others are noise. Weak embodiment theorists, for example, focus on our brains and the body as the focal point of cognitive theorizing. Everything else in the list is just incidental—noise in our theorizing. Strong embodiment theorists who ignore the role of social and cultural forces think of 1–5 and 8–10 as the materials from which we build cognitive theories. Notice that we're in the same area as when we introduced the tuning knob metaphor. The tuning dials give you theories, and distinguishing between signal and noise in understanding the mind tells you how to move the knobs.

Maybe you're throwing your hands up in the air at this point, "well, how do we tell which theory is right if we can't even agree on what's relevant for a theory about embodied minds?!?" That's a fair question. And be cool, because our answer is unsatisfying: the most we can do is do some philosophy and some science and figure out which theories offer the best kinds of explanations for as many things as we want explained.

The more you know: There's an image of our understanding of the world, known as **Neurath's Boat**. The idea is that we're building our conceptual scheme—our understanding of the world—as we're using it. Suppose every creature you've seen with fins swimming through the water is a fish. Now you learn about dolphins: they have fins and swim through the water, but unlike fish, they give live birth and are warm-blooded. You could say either, "wow, some fish are warm-blooded and give live birth!" or "wow, some animals that have fins and swim through the sea aren't fish!" How you make that decision informs your ideas about fish. You're making adjustments to your conceptual scheme as you're using it.

The image that Otto Neurath uses is that we're building our boats as we're sailing them. Part of our journey on our own Neurathian Boats is that we have to discern what seems relevant to us as we're building our ideas about the mind.

Over time, we make changes to our theories—sometimes they're big and sometimes they're small. Science is ultimately a collaborative effort—collaborating across communities as well as across time with those who have gone before. And if we're going to do some philosophy that works hand in hand with science, then we need to acknowledge that our best theories will change over time too. There are plenty of disagreements, to be sure. But (ideally) those disagreements challenge philosophers and scientists to develop better and better theories about the nature of the mind.

In Chapters 7 and 8, we'll look at some folks who consider the brain, the body, and our evolutionary history to be the signal and everything else to be noise. In Chapters 9 and 10, we consider some folks who think there's a little bit of signal in each of the above-mentioned influences on the mind.

Notes

1 In this chapter, we're using Clark and Chalmers' ideas in "The Extended Mind" as a way of motivating the distinction between weaker and stronger versions of embodiment. The picture we develop is not chronological but instead uses an exciting idea (extended mind) to develop differences among embodiment theorists. We think it makes for a compelling presentation and hope you do too. We'll also map out the theoretical landscape in this chapter. You don't need it in order to keep going with the book, but it's helpful for getting a sense of the nuances of the theories and the space of possibilities for developing ideas about embodiment.

2 What's the relationship between reliable coupling and the Parity Principle? In Clark and Chalmers's paper, the Parity Principle is used as a way to identify what is (and is not) part of the extended mind. Reliable coupling comes in later, in the example with Otto and Inga, as a reason to think the cases should be

regarded as the same sort of case (i.e., as part of the activity of going to the MoMA). The Parity Principle helps us pick out what parts of the world are part of the extended mind. Reliable coupling explains how those parts of the world connect with people and become part of their cognitive systems.

3 Richard Menary and John Sutton are among the initial advocates for this position. This is often described as **second-wave extended mind**. It's important to note that Parity and Complementarity aren't either-or claims. You could actually think they're both right! Sutton notes this in his work and we see it in Clark too. He says what holds extended systems together is "trust and glue."

4 If you're like us, you have to think about which to use: "complimentary" or "complementary." When there's an "i", you're saying something nice, like, "you have a lovely home!" When there's an "e", it's when one thing fits with another: "the shirt complements the suit nicely!" We'll be using the one with an "e".

5 Or blackboard if you're old school.

6 We're persnickety about phrasing this point because a lot of fruitless arguments have broken out because of a misstatement about Parity.

7 This is a key idea underlying **ecological psychology**, which we'll discuss later.

8 Professional philosophers often describe the features we're highlighting here as "4E cognition": embodied, embedded, extended, and enactive. We think it's better, pedagogically, to keep 4E lingo in the footnotes, and we'll reference it when appropriate.

9 Someone might protest that the mechanics of the spine don't convey information the way the eye does and, therefore, they're not properly part of our cognitive abilities. That's a fair objection, and one that many philosophers find compelling. The objection highlights a more fundamental question about investigating cognition: how do we decide what's important to include as we're thinking about cognition? The brain matters, for sure, but what about the peripheral nervous system or the hands? We'll discuss this some more in §6.4.

10 For conservatism in science, jump ahead to "The More You Know" in §7.2.

11 Often referred to as enactive perception, detailed in Alva Noë's book, *Action in Perception*).

12 These kinds of radios were called "tuned radio frequency receivers" They consisted of three dials for very precise pickup of radio waves.

13 The brain-in-a-vat thought experiment asks us to imagine that each of us is a brain in a vat of nutrients. Our brains are stimulated by a complicated machine connected to them through many electrodes. We *think* we're living, breathing humans wandering around the world, but *really* we're just brains in vats.

14 This is a view that might work well with certain kinds of **determinism**, something we'll explore in Chapter 12.

7

WEAK EMBODIED COGNITION

7.1 Chapter overview

Weak embodied cognition is characterized by commitment to some machinery of disembodiment, namely, representations. This is done by separating the structure and content of representations. A representation's structure reflects a sense modality (e.g., sight, smell) and thereby shapes how that representation is processed. A representational account of embodiment allows for smooth integration with a cognitivist account of emotion as well as first-wave extended mind (see Chapter 4).

7.2 Connecting to the jazz standard

We examined the question, "where does the mind end and the rest of the world begin?" in Chapter 4. One thing we landed on is that the mind doesn't end at the skull; it extends out into the world.

That's all fine and dandy, but for the mind to extend into the world, it has to go through the body. There are different ways of "going through the body." In this chapter, we're going to look at one way that's fairly minimal. The short version of the story is that we retain a lot of the machinery of representationalism (we covered this in Chapter 3; go ahead and flip back if you don't remember), but we find a way to work the body into the story. We'll see that by doing this, we get a way of connecting this kind of embodiment to the sort of extended mind that Clark and Chalmers offer.

DOI: 10.4324/9781003356622-9

7.3 Motivating weak embodied cognition

We saw in Chapter 3 that Hilary Putnam used some ideas from Alan Turing to describe the mind as a kind of computer.

But now we're in a pickle. Representationalism—in the weak sense we discussed in "the more you know" from §3.1—sees the mind as disembodied.[1] It's entirely possible to talk about representations, content, information, and mental processes without mentioning the body at all. Notice that we did it in Chapter 3 with George Miller and the limits of working memory. The senses are ways to get information into the mind, and the cognitive scientist is concerned with the information after it's input into the mind from the senses. How that information gets from the eyes and the ears to the mind is a question for biologists. Once that info gets to the mind, it's up to cognitive scientists to figure out what happens.

So now the big question: is it possible to have an embodied representationalism? Is there any way that we can hold on to the default position in cognitive science and philosophy of mind *and yet* still require reference to bodies? Alvin Goldman proposes a way.

7.4 Connecting representations and the body

Weak embodiment is the view that the body shapes our mental representations, which in turn affects their role in our thinking. Goldman, for example, says that some of our representations have "bodily formats." The body plays a role in cognition by affecting how the representation is formatted. How a representation is formatted affects how it is processed and its contribution to our thinking. Now, what is the evidence in favor of this position? We'll do some stage setting before delivering the evidence and arguments.

7.4.1 Transducers and the body

One possibility is to "translate" all references to the body into the language of computations and representations. We account for the influence of the body by connecting the body's processes with the mind's processes. And we make this connection by talking about bodily processes using the lingo of computations and representations. An analogy might help. Think about a record player for a moment. The big picture is that the record spins and sound comes out of the speaker. But how do grooves on a record turn into sounds from a speaker? There has to be a conversion or "translation." The vibrations from the needle have to be converted to an electric signal. Imagine this at a very abstract level:

vibrations → converter → electric signal → amp → speaker

The converter is responsible for the "translation," but how does the converter work? The short answer is that the converter is a **transducer.** This transducer is made up of a needle, magnets, and coils. These items convert the sound vibrations into an electric signal, which is then fed to the amp and speaker.

The important lesson for us is that there has to be *some kind of process by which signals of one kind are turned into signals of another.* In the case of record players, sound vibrations are turned into electrical signals by means of the transducer. So how does it work for minds and bodies?

The More You Know: You might be thinking to yourself, "Why do signals from the body have to be converted into signals to our minds?" Thinking through this will help illustrate a point about **philosophy of science**—which is just thinking philosophically about science.

One option is to just be a **dualist**: the body does what it does and the mind does what it does and they *somehow* interact. This is a well-represented position in the history of philosophy, most notably by René Descartes. Even so, it doesn't shed much light on the relationship between mind and body. So we have bodily signals, and mental signals but how they interact is a mystery.

Another option is to be an **eliminativist**. Eliminativism says that all of our talk about minds should be eliminated in favor of talk about brains. In other words, eliminativism says that psychology is a bad science that needs to be junked; neuroscience is the better science of human behavior. In the present context, eliminativism tells us that we can hold on to our theories about bodily functioning and integrate them into an understanding of the brain. In this case, there's no need for conversion or translation of bodily signals into mental ones. There's nothing but bodily signals.

We have a few options on the table that would let us avoid the translating step we've been discussing. So why bother with translating bodily processes into mental ones? Briefly, recall from §4.6.2 that science tends to be conservative—it changes slowly and tries to accommodate new information into existing theories instead of junking the existing theories entirely. Here, that means incorporating our discoveries about the body's role in our mental lives into our current theories about the mind. Our current theories about the mind say that we're basically computers, so conservatism in science requires that we translate findings about the body into the lingo of mental processes.

There are cells that are sensitive to things outside the body: light-sensitive ones, touch-sensitive ones, and sound-sensitive ones. When these things are simulated, they create electrical impulses that move to different parts of the brain. So what's happening here? One way to look at it is that the stimuli are *transduced* into electrical "information." That is, the stimuli are "converted" into information that the mind can process. Jerry Fodor (1983) argued that the mind/brain has transducers. Their job is to convert signals from the senses to information that can be processed in the mind. The outputs of those transducers are mental representations.

Now, as we saw "in §3.3.2", philosophers and psychologists distinguish between the representation as a vehicle for content and the content of the representations. So when we're trying to incorporate the influence of the body into mental processes, our first choice is between *vehicles* and *contents*. A thought's content is what the thought is about. So if the body shows up in the content of the thought, then the thought is about that bit of the body. When you step on a rusty nail and think, "Fiddle-dee-dee, that will require a tetanus shot,"[2] you are thinking about the pain in your foot.

So while the body can show up in the contents of our thoughts (i.e., we can think about our bodies and their parts), this isn't quite what embodied cognition advocates have in mind. When your hanger results in poor life choices—or at least being snarky with your co-workers—you're not thinking about your stomach. You're thinking about how their habit of taking excessively long bathroom breaks means you're left with more of the cleaning. Or maybe how infinitely annoying it is when they're clipping their nails at their desk.[3] What you're not thinking about is the rumbling in your stomach or the mild headache.

That means that we're left with the vehicle as the place to get the body into the cognitive system. This is precisely what Goldman proposes in several places (2011, 2014; Goldman and Vignemont 2009). Let's dig a little deeper into his proposal and why he makes the philosophical moves he does.

7.4.2 Modes of thought and perception

Don't overthink this one: you see with your eyes, you hear with your ears, and you smell with your nose. When you're perceiving the world, your perceptions are **modality**-specific. Visual perceptions come from your visual system; auditory perceptions come from your auditory system; **proprioceptive** perceptions come from your proprioceptive system. The mode of perception is a product of the system that produces the perception. If that's not clear, just remember: visual perceptions come from the visual system.

The More You Know: Proprioception is an unusual sense. It's awareness of your body's position in space. For instance, if you put your hand behind your back and hold up three fingers, you know you're holding up three fingers. You don't need to see your fingers to know that three of them are up. It turns out that proprioception is *really* important. A man named Ian Waterman lost all proprioception from the neck down and had trouble with everyday activities like walking or sitting upright.

But a lot of our thinking doesn't obviously come from any perceptual system: when we're doing a bit of mental math or trying to figure out why the car won't start, we aren't relying solely on perception. You might have to look at the engine to determine why the car won't start, but you still have to do a bit of thinking about what you see. That bit of thinking might rely on vision for inputs, but there's still some thinking to be done that isn't about what you immediately see. You have to think about what *should* be there or *should* be connected but isn't.

Another example is when you're imagining something. This is a kind of mental activity where you don't need any of your senses. You can close your eyes and imagine a warm sunny beach. You don't need to be looking at the beach in order to imagine it.

When you're thinking in this kind of way, the representations involved are **amodal**—it seems as though they aren't based in any specific sort of perceptual modality. So mental math doesn't depend on your auditory system like hearing a tree fall in the forest does. The representations involved in doing mental math are amodal; the representations involved with hearing the tree fall are modal. "Modal," in other words, means "specific to a mode of perception." And "amodal" means "not specific to a mode of perception."

We have two kinds of representations: modal and amodal. Most of our abstract thinking—the kind of thinking that Descartes put on a pedestal—seems amodal. So when you're thinking to yourself, "Why won't Janet shut up about her eight cats?" you're not using your hearing or vision or proprioception in any clear way. Still, your gnawing hunger is eating away at your patience for Janet.

This is how Goldman reframes the problem. Instead of asking, "How does the body affect the mind," he makes the question more precise: how can modal representations play a role in amodal thought?

Otto's workbook: Philosophers spend a lot of time refining questions. They do this because we have to ask good questions to get good answers. If our questions are vague, our answers will be too. What's an example where you had to figure out the right question to ask to get the kinds of answers you needed?

Goldman's argument is that what often *seem* to be amodal representations are *actually* modal representations. In other words, when you're thinking about what to have for dinner (for example), that might seem amodal on the face of it, but it actually involves some of the body's perceptual systems. He calls these kinds of representations **bodily formats:** thoughts whose vehicles are modal even though their contents are not. A "format" is a representational system with a distinctive array of contents, processes, and structures.[4] He offers two lines of evidence. We'll go through them one at a time.

7.4.2.1 Lakoff and Johnson on conceptual structures

Let's think for a moment about how we talk about things. We often don't talk literally. We say things like "I've been feeling kinda down lately" and "everything's coming up Milhouse!" When something is unsettled, we say "that's up in the air." When an event wasn't worthwhile, we say "well, *that* was a waste of time."

It's a little odd, isn't it, to talk about feeling bad in terms of direction (i.e., down), or time as a resource that can be used poorly. I can waste perfectly good food by letting it rot on the counter. But time isn't a concrete thing. How is time *wasted*? Also: I *spend* a lot of time fixing my car; but again, time isn't currency; how can I spend time?

In these cases and many others, we talk about one thing in terms of another. That is, we use *metaphors* in our talk. Metaphors are *everywhere*. Think about as simple an exchange as:

Bill: *How's it going?*
Ted: *It's going ok.*

We understand Bill to be asking Ted about his current state of affairs: his mood, recent notable events, his living conditions, etc. But what is "it" and how does it go anywhere? It's all metaphors.

George Lakoff and Mark Johnson developed **conceptual metaphor theory** as a way to explain a wide range of phenomena in language and thought. The core idea (another metaphor!) is that language and thought are largely metaphorical. Our concepts are structured as metaphors; that is, we have a basic stock of concepts and we use this basic stock of metaphorical concepts for understanding the world around us.

Let's use an example: HAPPY IS UP. Think about some of the ways we talk about happiness. "I'm on top of the world," "I'm on Cloud 9," "She's in high spirits." We think about happiness as being up and sadness as being down. So where do our concepts UP and DOWN come from?

First, note that "up" and "down" are meaningful for us because of our bodies—up is whatever is above our heads and down is below our feet. Our bodies have a spatial orientation to the world. There is a definite front and back to humans; an obvious top and bottom. We can bring out our orientation to the world by means of a thought experiment. Just imagine a single hydrogen atom floating in space. One single atom floating in the vast emptiness of space. Which side is the front and which is the back? What is on top of or beneath this atom? Any choice is as good as any other. There is no significant orientation for this single atom—you can pick any side and call it the front or the back or the top or bottom. But humans aren't like this. We have a front and a back; a top and a bottom. We are spatially oriented to the world.

Now, why is happy *up* and sad *down*? Lakoff and Johnson speculate that our physical posture often droops when we're sad. Also, when we're sick, we often lie down. And being dead is about as down (physically) as you can get. In contrast, we stand tall when we're happy. When we're healthy, we're upright and moving around.

Now, whether *this* explanation is right doesn't matter for our purposes. There could be plenty of other reasons why we associate HAPPY with UP and SAD with DOWN. Heck, it's even logically possible to associate HAPPY with DOWN and SAD with UP.

> **Otto's Workbook**: Write a very short story (like, ten sentences) about someone being happy using the metaphor HAPPY IS UP. Now rewrite that story using the metaphor HAPPY IS DOWN. What was it like to use that alternative metaphor?

So what *does* matter for us when we're thinking about conceptual metaphor theory and embodiment? First, that there are these associations: we do in fact associate HAPPY with UP. Second, UP and DOWN are meaningful for us because of our bodily orientation. It's because we have a head and two feet that concepts like UP and DOWN have any meaning at all. Again, if we were point particles floating in empty space, "up" and "down" would be meaningless. This suggests that our concepts are partly grounded in our bodily experiences in the world. Our concepts are what they are because of the bodies and orientations to the world that we have. HAPPY can be UP because we have the kinds of bodies situated in a world for which UP is meaningful. Even if our single hydrogen atom were to become sentient, UP would fail to be meaningful for this atom—there's no meaningful sense of up or down for it.

What Goldman takes away from conceptual metaphor theory is that many—perhaps all—of our concepts are grounded in the body. The body has to appear in either the content or the structure. It can't be in virtue of their contents. The metaphors TIME IS MONEY or HAPPY IS UP don't show up in the contents of thoughts like "I'm wasting my time" or "She's in high spirits today." So the metaphors that govern our thinking *don't do so in virtue of their contents*. Since metaphorical thinking doesn't happen in virtue of the content, it must happen in virtue of the thought's structure, the thought's vehicle. We can write out the argument like this:

1 Most of our abstract thinking uses metaphors;
2 Metaphors are grounded in our bodies;
3 Therefore, most of our abstract thinking is grounded in our bodies;
4 If most of our abstract thinking is grounded in our bodies, then there is a representational system that accounts for the role of the body in abstract thinking that does not involve the body;
5 Therefore, there is a representational system that accounts for the role of the body in abstract thinking that does not involve the body.

Let's walk through the logic of the argument.

1 Lines 1 and 2 are restatements of conceptual metaphor theory;
2 Line 3 follows from 1 and 2 by replacing "metaphors" in line 1 with the whole of line 2;
3 Line 4 combines conceptual metaphor theory and the cognitive scientific theory of representational systems (aka "formats");
4 Line 5 comes from lines 3 and 4 (this is the argument pattern **modus ponens**).

Our thoughts are about all kinds of things; however, since most of our thinking is metaphorical and the metaphors are grounded in our embodied experiences, the body shapes a lot of our thinking.

7.4.2.2 Anderson on neural reuse

Goldman's next piece of evidence comes from Michael Anderson's work on **neural reuse**. The work can get somewhat technical, but we'll keep it to what's relevant for Goldman's argument.

There is a long tradition in neuroscience that parts of the brain—and even certain kinds of neurons—are devoted to particular tasks. That's to say: different parts of the brain are dedicated to different tasks. This started to gain widespread acceptance when Paul Broca published his research on his subject, "Tan." The patient, a man named Louis Victor Leborgne, experienced a stroke at a young age that damaged part of his left **frontal lobe**. He could only produce one sound: "tan." Leborgne could nonetheless *understand* spoken language. He would respond to questions with "tan tan" of varying inflection and would gesture.[5] After Leborgne's death, Broca autopsied him and found the damage to his frontal lobe.

Not too long after Leborgne's death, another patient at the hospital where Broca worked—Lazare Lelong—had lost the ability to say anything except for five words: "yes," "no," "three," "always," and his name. After Lelong died, Broca took a peek at his brain too. He found a lesion to a region that largely overlapped with the damaged region of Leborgne.

The lesson from Broca is that parts of the brain are *specialized* in their functions. Neuroscientists call this **localization**: certain functions, like vision, speech, face recognition, etc., are located in specific regions of the brain. If you knock out those regions, you knock out the associated function. This is often taken to lead to a **modular** view of brain function: the brain is constituted by sets of neurons that have specific functions.

This seems like a fairly widespread and commonsense view—every mental function is associated with a part of the brain. And it actually matches the computational and representational view of mind really well: different parts of the brain store different kinds of representations and different parts of the brain are dedicated to different kinds of processing. But Anderson's work complicates this picture. What he and his team found is that many parts of the brain are recruited for many different sorts of tasks. We're going to take this step-by-step.

Let's put some pressure on the modular view. If the modular view is right, then very different kinds of activities would involve different (presumably non-overlapping) parts of the brain. For example, suppose kicking a ball involved region A of the brain, and imagining what to make for dinner involved region B. Kicking a ball and imagining what to make for dinner are very different kinds of activities. Since A and B are the areas responsible for kicking a ball and imagining dinner, A and B must also not have overlapping parts. (Remember, there are different sets of neurons for different activities on the modular view.)

However, this isn't what we find at all! It turns out that different activities recruit overlapping areas of the brain. Anderson's work says that we can't point to one part of the brain and say, "this is where imagination happens." Let's first talk about a few specific studies pointing to this conclusion. Then we'll go into the general lesson for weak embodied cognition.

First, Friedemann Pulvermüller (2005) argues that fMRI data show that action-related words activate areas of the brain that are related to the words being uttered in addition to areas of the brain associated with language. "Pick" and "kick," for example, activate parts of the brain that are typically associated with language comprehension. But hearing "pick" also activates parts of the **motor cortex** associated with hand movement. And the same is true for "kick" except for parts of the motor cortex associated with leg movement. What this means is that understanding the meaning of the word involves parts of the brain traditionally associated with language comprehension *but also* parts of the brain associated with movement. He calls these "action-perception circuits."

The More You Know: What's the big deal with the fact that some words activate parts of the brain associated with bodily movement? Suppose for a moment that action and cognition were completely separate processes, as the representational and computational view of mind supposes. If they're completely separate processes, then we wouldn't expect to see any overlap in parts of the brain associated with those processes. Why would *that* be the case? The main reason is that we'd be left with an awkward explanatory situation. We'd have to come up with a good story for why the mental processes are distinct but the neural processes aren't.

Now, you might think to yourself, "Can't there be *some* overlap in neural regions? Why would that be a problem for the modular view?" You're right that the modular view can say that there is *some* overlap between neural regions. This is the difference between a weak modular view and a strong modular view. The strong view says that there is *no* overlap. The weak view says there is *some* overlap.

So would a weak modular view be compatible with the idea of embodied cognition? Yes! Some embodiment theorists want to hold on to ideas about modularity *and* that some cognitive processes are embodied. These folks endorse a weak modular view. Other scientists and philosophers want to ditch the modular view entirely.

Second, psychologists have discovered a phenomenon called the **action sentence compatibility effect**. The idea is that there is an interaction between the meanings of our sentences and the actions we perform. Arthur Glenberg and Michael Kaschak (2002) use Lakoff and Johnson's work as a springboard for their own ideas. They hypothesized that understanding a sentence would be easier if readers were performing an action that was similar to one implied by the sentence. An example will make this easier. Suppose we tell you, "Give the cookie to your sister." Giving is an action that involves moving something away from the body. So even though we never explicitly say that giving involves an action of moving away from the body, it's implicit in the meaning of "give." For a similar idea, consider "Take the keys out of the door." Taking has as part of its meaning an action of bringing something closer to you. Just think: you don't *take* something by making it farther away from you.

Glenberg and Kaschak explored this hypothesis by having participants judge whether a sentence was nonsense or not. Sentences included "You took the pizza" and "You delivered the pizza," as well as nonsense sentences like "You gave the earring Susan." Subjects would indicate whether the sentence made sense or not by hitting a button that was either *further* from them or *closer* to them. So you can imagine two conditions: when the action and the sentence meaning *matched* (closer button and "take"; further button and "give") or when the action and sentence meaning *mismatched* (closer button and "give"; further button and "take"). It turns out that people were a lot faster in judging whether the sentence made sense or not in the *matching* conditions as opposed to the *mismatching* conditions. That is, when reading "You gave the earring Susan," people judged it as nonsense more quickly when the button was further away instead of being closer to them. It seems that sentence comprehension and action somehow interact with one another.

The results for both Pulvermüller and Glenberg and Kaschak suggest that our language and motor systems affect one another. They aren't isolated from each other. One way to make sense of these results is that each of those parts of the brain is active in the same kinds of activities. Most importantly, it is that language production and comprehension overlaps with the action "centers" of the brain.

Anderson's neural reuse theory explains this by saying that the same brain areas are used in both kinds of activities, but with different connections between each other and with other areas of the brain. In other words, neural reuse predicts that different areas of the brain are at work in all kinds of activities. There are very few (if any) areas devoted to specific tasks. So it makes sense, according to neural reuse theory, that language and motor systems affect one another—they're often using the same sets of neurons!

So how does Goldman use neural reuse to make sense of weak embodied cognition? The argument runs roughly like this:

1 Some "higher" cognitive processes (e.g., language) depend on some of the same brain circuits as action processes;
2 If some "higher" processes depend on action processes, then those processes require bodily formats;
3 Therefore, some "higher" processes require bodily formats.

The More You Know: Why is "higher" in scare quotes? Since at least Plato in the Western tradition, philosophers distinguish between our intellectual, cognitive capacities and our emotional and physical ones. The intellectual capacities are often thought of as better or superior to our physical ones—probably because it's what makes us different from other animals. But thinking about our intellectual capacities as "better than" our physical or emotional ones is a value judgment that we're not willing to make at this moment. It seems to us that in some cases, being able to fight a wild animal can be a superior skill to solving differential equations. Nonetheless, the lingo is what it is, and we'll go along with it while trying our best to bring out the implicit assumptions about the nature of mind and body.

A related point is that **representation-hungry problems**—that is, cognitive processes (like doing some mental math or planning a vacation) that seem to require mental representations as part of an adequate explanation—are often "higher" cognitive processes. Identifying the consequences of some action is a "higher" cognitive process and seems to require mental representations.[6] We'll have more to say about representation-hungry problems in Chapters 10 and 12.

And again, the logic of the argument:

- Line 1 is a restatement of Anderson's neural reuse hypothesis;
- Line 2 is a way of talking about bodily formats;
- Line 3 follows from lines 1 and 2 by *modus ponens*.

Let's focus on Line 2 for a moment. We're interested in the neural circuits themselves, not in the meaning of anything. We distinguished between content and form: neural connections are firmly on the "form" side. There might be some content or information in patterns of neural activation, but we're not concerned with that. We're focusing *only* on the neural structure: the connections among neurons and regions of the brain.

But this means that language and "higher" cognition involve modal representations! "Higher" cognition is produced, in part, by action systems, and representations in action systems are modal. (Why? A command like "run to the pizzeria" has to be issued in a format such that it can be employed by the neuromuscular system of the legs.) And showing that "higher" cognition is modal is exactly what Goldman set out to argue.

7.5 Summarizing Goldman's view

Let's do a quick recap of Goldman's weak embodied cognition.

He thinks about thinking in terms of representations and computations. In that way, he has a lot in common with Noam Chomsky and Alan Turing. So how does the body shape thought? It does so by affecting the structure of the representation. While classical representationalists think about "higher" cognition as *amodal*—that is, not dependent on any particular sense modality—Goldman argues that "higher" cognition is *modal*. So our concepts about happiness are shaped by our bodily orientation to the world and the fact that being upright is good (i.e., not sick, tired, or dead). My thought, "Fido is chasing a squirrel" doesn't only activate pieces of my frontal lobe but also my motor cortex. Squirrel-chasing thoughts are connected, by way of overlapping patterns of neural activity, with squirrel-chasing behavior.

We call this "weak" embodied cognition because it doesn't require us to ditch or overhaul the default concepts of representations and computations. The body is incorporated into an account of cognition, but only by way of shaping representations' structures. Goldman's weak embodied cognition isn't an entirely disembodied account of the mind, but it's about as close as one can get to keeping the default concepts and yet still attending to the role of the body in cognition.

7.6 Emotions

Emotions have a weird place in philosophy. On the one hand, they have a mental aspect to them. Imagine you're angry with Karen for taking *your* piece of cake from the office fridge. You're angry with Karen because you believe that she's the one who took the cake. Now, if you later learn that it wasn't Karen but rather Chad who took the cake, then you are no longer angry at Karen but rather at Chad. So your anger is responsive to your beliefs about the world. Your anger has a mental aspect to it.

But your anger also has a physical aspect. You feel different when you're angry. Perhaps you get hot under the collar (literally), or you clench your jaw. Either way, there's some kind of physiological change when you are angry.

Emotions are often thought of as a kind of halfway place between mind and body. They have long been discussed in philosophy. Aristotle believed they were a crucial part of explaining why we act as we do and also that shaping our emotional responses is crucial for living a good life. Descartes thought of emotions largely in a physiological way. They are part of the story to explain how the body moves, but they didn't play a big role in his theories about mind and cognition. **David Hume** flipped the order of operations, describing reason as a "slave" to the passions.

So how might a weak embodiment theorist incorporate emotions into an account of embodiment? While he more strongly identifies with the cognitivist tradition (that we discussed in Chapter 3), Ronald de Sousa offers a view in his book *The Rationality of Emotions*. This overview will gloss over *a lot* of details. If this piques your interest, go take a look. There are two key points for us. The first is that emotions indeed have a felt, bodily component to them. This is a result of the biology we've inherited from our evolutionary history: it's *really* useful to have your adrenaline pumping when you're afraid. So the feelings characteristic of anger, sadness, joy, and so on are part of what it is to have that emotion. The second point is that the target of our anger or any other emotion is a mental representation.[7] You can believe that the sky is blue and that means you have a mental representation whose content is *the sky is blue*. Similarly, you can be happy that the sky is blue and that means you have a mental representation whose content is, *the sky is blue*. De Sousa's strategy is to treat emotions like other intentional states like belief and desire.

This is a *weak* embodiment because de Sousa pulls together two distinct elements: emotions' bodily feel and the target of emotions as mental representations. There is a bodily part to the story. Our emotions have a feel to them that is the result of our biology. There is also the cognitive part that emotions are directed at mental representations.

7.7 Extending Goldman's view

Now that we've covered Goldman's view, let's connect it with another element from the Jazz Standard discussed in Chapter 4.

Goldman's view is a kind of functionalism—recall that functionalism defines mental states in terms of their inputs and outputs. Goldman adds that the structures of some of those mental states are informed by bodily states. Remember also that the variety of extended mind we find in Clark and Chalmers (1998) is a kind of extended functionalism. Something counts as part of the extended cognitive system if it works in a way that, if it happened inside the head, it would be counted as cognitive. Otto's notebook is part of his cognitive system because it works like parts of Inga's brain. So the big question is: can we make weak embodied cognition into a kind of extended mind theory?[8] The answer, unsurprisingly, is: it depends. Let's go through our options.

First, insofar as weak embodied cognition is a kind of functionalism, we can apply the arguments from Clark and Chalmers. Remember the Parity Principle: if something outside the head works like mechanisms inside the head, and if that something outside the head would be considered part of the cognitive system if it were inside the head, then that something outside the head is part of the cognitive system. Someone who thinks weak embodied cognition gets things right could take the Otto thought experiment on board without a problem.[9] Otto's notebook holds readily available information that's trusted upon retrieval, and the same can be said for a representation of the same information inside someone's skull.

But there's a wrinkle: for weak embodied cognition, some of our mental representations are structured by the body, which means that only bodies like ours could have mental representations like ours. Extended mind theory (when thought of as an extended functionalism—see Chapter 4 for details) endorses a kind of functionalism in which the underlying matter is irrelevant. All that matters is the inputs and outputs. So weak embodied cognition says that the underlying matter is relevant and extended mind theory says it's not.

Is there any way we can get past this? Here are a few ideas:

1 Weak embodied cognition says that there are still some mental representations that are amodal—that is, not structured with bodily inputs. So perhaps it's only for *some* mental processes that the underlying matter is relevant. That would leave space to argue that those mental processes for which the underlying matter is irrelevant are the kinds of processes that can be outside the head and yet still part of the cognitive system.
2 An extended mind theorist could point out that processes and representations outside the body have to be able to fit with our physical abilities. Otto's notebook, for instance, would be useless if the script were too small to read or written in invisible ink. So in a sense, processes and representations outside the head are already structured by the body: they have to be usable by organisms like us with our physical abilities.

So there you have it: a weak embodiment theorist could bring extended mind theory on board without too many snags. This brief back-and-forth doesn't settle the matter altogether, but it might give you some food for thought about how to unite them.

7.8 Conclusion

If you find yourself impressed with both a computational view of cognition, but still want to make room for the body, weak embodiment is up your alley. You even have some fairly powerful conceptual resources not offered by computationalism on its own—namely, conceptual metaphor theory and neural reuse. This provides you with a way to hold on to a fairly traditional view of the mind and still make some room for the body.

You don't need to make huge adjustments to your conceptual scheme. You can even give an account of the nature of emotions!

The arguments in favor of weak embodiment hinge on interpreting data from neuroscience and cognitive science in a conservative way: bringing the new data on board without making huge adjustments to the basic theoretical framework. This is a bit of having your cake and eating it too: you get the conceptual resources of a well-developed theory about the mind as well as the additional resources of embodiment, albeit constrained by the background theory.

Notes

1 As a reminder: the weak sense of disembodiment is that psychological explanations are independent of biological explanations. We—scientists and laypersons—can provide psychological explanations for behavior without referring to biological or neuroscientific explanations.
2 *The Simpsons*, season 3, episode 16, "Bart the Lover."
3 These examples are completely fabricated and in no way have any connection to the lives of the authors.
4 The idea of a format comes from the modularity hypothesis that we introduced above.
5 If you're a *Simpsons* fan, think of "Who Shot Mr. Burns? Part Two" (season 7, episode 1). After waking in the hospital after being shot, all Mr. Burns can say is "Homer Simpson" with various inflections.
6 There are some interesting questions we can ask here: are all "higher" cognitive processes representation-hungry? Are all representation-hungry tasks also "higher" cognitive processes? Is there something about "higher" cognitive processes that requires representations? Is there something about representations that makes them particularly apt for explaining "higher" cognitive processes? We don't have the time or space to go any deeper, but we think these are interesting questions worth thinking about.
7 This is a bit misleading. De Sousa actually holds that the targets of our emotions are **propositions.** Propositions are whatever it is that "the cat is white" and "el gato esta blanca" have in common. They are often thought of as what sentences mean. There are some subtle differences with respect to propositions and mental representations. One big one is that propositions and mental representations are individuated in different ways. That is: what makes one mental representation different from another isn't the same as what makes one proposition different from another. See the entry on "propositions" in the *Stanford Encyclopedia of Philosophy* for more details. Additionally, as we'll see in § 9.4.5, this isn't the only view of emotions that philosophers discuss.
8 You can endorse weak embodiment and not extended mind. The weak-embodiment-non-extended-mind person says, "Yeah the body shapes cognitive processes but all the machinery is inside the body."
9 Notice we used "could take on board." Lots of folks who prefer weak embodied cognition because it is less radical than other varieties of embodied cognition are also reluctant to endorse extended mind theory. Fred Adams is someone like this. What we want to point out in this section is that there are ways of understanding weak embodied cognition and extended mind such that they're compatible.

8

OBJECTIONS TO WEAK EMBODIED COGNITION

8.1 Chapter overview

In the previous chapter, we looked at weak embodied cognition and reasons in favor of it. In this chapter, we consider reasons against weak embodied cognition. The criticisms can be lumped into three categories: weak embodied cognition inherits problems with representationalism, weak embodied cognition is not radical enough, and weak embodied cognition is too radical.

8.2 Ways to raise concerns about weak embodied cognition

Goldman bills his weak embodied cognition as a moderate view. On the one hand, he wants to keep as much of representationalist cognitive science as possible. So he's happy bringing a bunch of related concepts on board, but separates them from a disembodied mind. On the other hand, he wants to show how the mind is embodied but doesn't want to take on theories about the mind that are so radical as to exclude the possibility of appealing to representations altogether. So his proposed middle ground is to incorporate embodiment into the structure of mental representations.

This characterization offers three ways of criticizing weak embodied cognition. First, we can take issue with representationalism. Second, we can show how the account fails to be radical enough. Third, we can look at how weak embodied cognition ends up being *too* radical and requiring us to abandon some otherwise common-sense ideas about mind.

DOI: 10.4324/9781003356622-10

8.3 Concerns with representationalism in weak embodied cognition

If you look back at Chapter 3, you'll find three major arguments against representationalism. They are:

1. Experiencing ourselves: the body is both subject and object, but representationalist views have a hard time accommodating this observation;
2. Concept of mind: our very concept of mind includes the body;
3. Symbol grounding: it's a mystery how our thoughts get to have the meanings they have.

Let's see how weak embodied cognition fares with each of these.

8.3.1 Experiencing ourselves

Can weak embodiment account for ourselves as subjects? Recall the phenomenon of double sensation: when you touch your palm with the index finger of the opposite hand, your body is an object that is being touched (your palm) and also a subject that is doing the touching (your finger). If minds are disembodied, then the body is always an object and never a subject. Your mind is always the subject.

Recall how the body gets into the mechanisms of cognition: through structuring representations. The body is then folded into the mind as part of the cognitive machinery. That is, the body helps with the activity of the mind; the role it plays is in the mind doing what it does. The body is part of the subject, but in an indirect way. The body is capable of being a subject only as it contributes to the structure of representations, which are then manipulated, stored, etc.

So can weak embodiment accommodate double sensation? As with so many things, it depends. We can distinguish between two senses of the body as subject: directly and indirectly. For the body to be a subject directly is to say that the subject is the body itself. Some older terminology for this comes from medieval philosophy, in particular Thomas Aquinas. Aquinas describes people as ensouled bodies.[1] Our modern version might be *minded bodies*. The expression refers to the fact that it's not that minds are "housed" in bodies but rather that bodies are "suffused" by mind.[2] Being a subject *indirectly* is more like Descartes's analogy of the sailor in the ship. We experience our bodies, but it's through representations. There is a mind and it receives input from sensory receptors.

The more you know: In philosophy, when we say that one thing is related to or affects another, we can distinguish between that relationship being direct (or immediate) and indirect (or mediate). For example, John Locke's view of perception held that we never perceive the world directly. We perceive the world indirectly, by means of ideas and images. You don't really see the mug but rather you have a percept of the mug. **Thomas Reid**, by contrast, argued that we perceive the mug directly, without the intervention of representations.

If being a subject means that the body has to be involved in *some* way, then yes: weak embodied cognition can accommodate the body as a feeling subject. The body is involved *indirectly* in perceiving the body as an object. When you touch your hand with your finger, then the experiencing subject—the mind—is receiving input through the palm of an object coming into contact with it. The object in this case just happens to be your finger. You can do the same thing with your finger—it transmits inputs about coming into contact with something (which happens to be your palm).

But if being a subject means that the body has to be involved directly, then no: weak embodied cognition cannot accommodate the body as a feeling subject. As we've described it, weak embodiment traffics in representations. Direct involvement of the body in subjectivity means that it's the minded body that is experiencing the sensation. When you touch your hand, you're not interacting with any intermediary—that is, no mental representations. Your experience is in your hands. Thinking and perception involve the brain but aren't reducible to it. It's the body as a whole that's involved in thinking and perception.

8.3.2 Concept of mind

Some good news: we finally have a clear answer! Weak embodied cognition *cannot* (easily) rebut the argument against disembodiment we saw in Chapter 3. That's because the argument that our concept of mind includes the concept of a body requires fleshy, sweaty, smelly bodies,[3] not just their influence on mental representations. So *if* you're convinced by Strawson's and Ryle's ideas, then you're probably not going to be too impressed with weak embodied cognition.[4]

8.3.3 Symbol grounding

This one turns out to be kind of tricky. Recall that the problem with symbol grounding is that there's no obvious way for thoughts to get their meanings. It can't come from other thoughts (like how words get their meanings from us), and it seems unusual to say it's just a fact about minds that our thoughts have the meanings they do.

At first, you might think that weak embodied cognition can handle symbol grounding because thoughts get their contents (in part) from their structure. That is, the bodily formatting of mental representations is part of how our thoughts get to have the meanings they have. An example might help. Recall that we think of HAPPY as being up and SAD as being down. Our concept of happiness is what it is in part because of how our bodies are oriented in the world. When we think about happiness as feeling elated or like walking in sunshine, this is because we are upright when we're in states of good health and well-being. So thoughts about happiness are what they are, in part, because of our bodies. This presents a way to address symbol grounding. Where do our thoughts get their contents? From our bodies.

But there are two lingering concerns. First, notice a key modifier in our description of how the body affects the contents of thought: "in part." This is because there are other debates about the nature of our thoughts, debates whose resolutions can have an effect on how we think about the body and mental contents. For example, are our concepts standalone entities or do their meanings shape one another? That is, can I have a concept like CAT all on its own or do I need other concepts like MAMMAL or ALLERGIES in order for my CAT concept to be what it is? This is the debate between **atomism** and **holism**. If it turns out that holism is true, then it's not just our bodies that determine the contents of our thoughts. It's other thoughts too. Therefore, it seems like the body has a diminishing role to play in what grounds our thoughts.

Otto's workbook: Holism is sometimes described as a "web," most notably by the philosopher **Willard Quine**. Draw a web of belief for the concept HAPPINESS. What other concepts would you connect to this concept?

The second lingering concern is that, according to Goldman, some thoughts are amodal. He doesn't give us too many hints, but we can imagine that thoughts about very abstract things like logic or imaginary numbers would be amodal. Imaginary numbers, for example, involve the square roots of negative numbers. In case your last math class was quite some time ago, (nonimaginary) squared numbers can never be negative: -5×-5 is 25, not -25. The imaginary number $5i$ is the square root of -25. Imaginary numbers are a construct that enables mathematicians to explore new ideas. While they turn out to be useful in engineering and physics, you'd have to tell a pretty inventive story to explain how imaginary numbers come from our bodily orientation in the world.

8.4 Not radical enough

Embodied cognition, as it was conceived by some of the 20th century's leading lights, was intended to be a view of the mind that departs substantially from representational views. Let's explore why and use that as a springboard to develop a criticism of weak embodied cognition.[5]

Recall two major empirical points that Goldman makes in developing his position: conceptual metaphor theory and neural reuse. Conceptual metaphor theory says that our concepts are based (in part) on our bodily orientation to the world—just keep coming back to the "HAPPY is UP" metaphor. Neural reuse says that there are very few (if any) specialized regions of the brain—the overlapping bits are involved in both activity and language, for instance—and this best explains why some cognitive tasks are shaped by behaviors.

Julian Kiverstein, in his criticisms of Goldman, points out that neural reuse seems to require a stronger reading on embodied cognition than Goldman allows. To see Kiverstein's objections, we'll need to make a detour into sandwich country.

There's a model of perception, thinking, and acting that we've seen before (described in Chapter 3). We perceive parts of the world. These perceptions are passed along into cognitive processing before issuing an action. I see a glass of water, form the belief that a glass of water is nearby and that I want the water, and then walk towards it. Schematically, it is perception → cognition → action. Susan Hurley calls this the "sandwich model" of cognition. Cognition is sandwiched between perception and action. Now, in order to have a cognition sandwich, you need three distinct elements: perception, cognition, and action—just like you need one slice of bread, some peanut butter, and a second slice of bread to make a sandwich. And just as you can examine each slice of bread and the peanut butter independently of one another, you can examine perception, cognition, and action independently of one another.

Representational views of mind often presuppose the sandwich model of cognition.

> **Otto's workbook**: Explain how representational views of mind often presuppose the sandwich model of cognition.

The argument, then, is this:

1 If representational views of mind are right, then the sandwich model of cognition is right;
2 The sandwich model of cognition is wrong;
3 Therefore, representational views of mind are wrong.

Premise 1 follows from how we've described representationalism and the sandwich model. Premise 2 comes from some scientific considerations (which we're about to go into). And the conclusion follows by *modus tollens*.

So premise 2 is the big one. Why think the sandwich model is wrong? Two reasons. The first consideration is a broad one that we'll end up talking about a bit more in the next chapter: perception is for action. When our ancient forebears climbed out of the muck, evolved over millions of years, and finally developed into humans with anxiety and stomach issues, they had to make sure they weren't killed in the process. They had to be able to perceive threats and respond accordingly. If they couldn't do this, they shuffled off their mortal coil in a very unpleasant way. The conclusion is that perception had to have evolved for action.

The second consideration goes back to Anderson's neural reuse theory. Recall that cognitive activities like remembering or language use involve lots of different parts of the brain, including parts associated with movement. There are no modules in the brain for language use, memory, or vision. Lots of parts are caught up in lots of activities. So there is no basis in the brain for dividing up perception, cognition, and action! That is, there are no divisions in brain activity that correspond to the sandwich model of cognition. This gives us a really good reason to think that the sandwich model is wrong, especially if you think that how the brain works gives us some insight into how the mind works.

In conclusion, the very data Goldman appeals to in order to make his case for weak embodied cognition demands a much more radical view of embodiment. And since Goldman's view is driven in large part by the scientific evidence, weak embodied cognition doesn't have much to stand on.

8.5 Too radical

While Kiverstein argued that weak embodied cognition wasn't radical enough, some hard-line disembodiment theorists might argue that it's *too* radical. How? It all comes down to **multiple realizability**. We mentioned it in passing in § 3.1 when we talked about consciousness being realized in silicon chips or neural tissue, and now we need some more details.

To say that a state or process is "multiply realizable" is to say that different kinds of physical things can be in that state or perform that process.[6] For example, take the process of sewing. A person with needle and thread can sew, and so can someone with a sewing machine. There are now even autonomous, industrial robots that sew. The activity of sewing is multiply realizable by different sorts of things. From here on, we'll talk about "states" and "systems" instead of "things."

One of the central ideas behind multiple realizability is functionalism. We mentioned this in Chapter 2. It thinks about minds in terms of input-output systems. You put in perceptions, beliefs, and desires on one end and get behavior out on the other. It might not surprise you to know that the computational theory of mind introduced in Chapter 3 is a functionalist view. How? Because it doesn't matter *what* is doing the computations, there just has to be *something* doing them. The key to functionalism is that mental states are defined in terms of their functions, and the matter that has the mental states—that *realizes* the mental states—doesn't really matter. Brains can believe that 2+2=4, and so can suitably sophisticated machines and aliens. Their beliefs are all the same because they have the same (or very similar) functional profile. They all have the same (or very similar) inputs and outputs.

Side quest: One big obstacle for functionalism[7] is giving an explanation of **qualia**—the what-it's-likeness of our experience—in terms of their physical realizers. Consider this argument from Frank Jackson (1986), first formulated by Nicholas Maxwell (1966). Imagine a cognitive scientist in a black-and-white lab—everything they do and see is in shades of gray. There's nothing wrong with their vision, it's just that the world around them has been constructed to be in black and white. Imagine further that this scientist has been in this lab their whole life—growing up, eating, and sleeping there—and that they know everything there is to know about how vision works. They know all about the neural mechanisms and have a totally worked out theory about computationalism and vision. Now, suppose one day this scientist leaves the lab and sees the blue sky, the green grass, the yellow-and-black of a goldfinch. Does our scientist learn anything new? Absolutely! They learn what it's like to perceive red, green, yellow, and black. But our cognitive scientist knew everything there was to know about the neuroscience and cognitive science of vision. So the neuroscience and cognitive science of vision don't tell us everything there is to know about vision. There are also qualia: the what-it's-likeness of experience.

Not everyone agrees with the conclusion. **David Lewis**, for example, argues that the scientist doesn't learn a new *fact*. Rather, she learns a new *ability*: seeing and imagining what colored things look like. (Note that this appeals to the knowledge-that and knowledge-how distinction we introduced in §6.2.3.) But abilities can be completely described by neuroscience: the sciences of the brain will be able to tell us what the brain is doing when anyone performs an action. So there's no mysterious "qualia," no unexplainable fact, that the scientist learns. So what do you think? Do you think the scientist learns something new? What is it they learn (if anything)—a fact or how to do something? Is learning what a goldfinch looks like similar to learning how to ride a bike? Or that 5+7=12?

Functionalism was, and still is, the dominant framework in philosophy of mind, in part because representationalism is so entrenched in psychology and cognitive science. It's hard to overstate just how much research takes functionalist views of mind for granted. Whenever you hear something about mental representations or conscious machines, these presume that functionalism (or something very much like it) is right.

Some hard-nosed representationalists can complain that weak embodied cognition is too radical. How? Remember that weak embodied cognition claims that for some of our mental representations, the structure is informed by our bodies. Let's use Goldman's label of "bodily formats" for talking about these sorts of representations. So if weak embodied cognition is right, then bodily formats can only be handled by humans with human bodies, which suggests that functionalism is false. Functionalism claims that the underlying matter realizing a mental process doesn't matter; weak embodied cognition says it does.

"But couldn't we just build a machine that's just like a human body?" you might be wondering. Let's think about the details of this proposal. Our machine would have to have a body shaped just like ours so it can interact in the world just as we do. After this, the details of the proposal start to get a little fuzzy. If the machine interacts with its environment as we do, how similar to us *internally* does that machine have to be? Does it have to have the same internal organs, or could it have a very different internal structure? If the same, then that pushes our questions back a step: do those machine organs have to be made up of the same kind of stuff as our organs? If different, we might reasonably ask, "if the machine looks human but is internally different, how much do we want to say that its body is enough like ours to have representations like ours?"

At this point, it's hard to say much more—we're moving beyond what we know and speculating about machines that are so similar to humans that they might think just like us. At this point, we'll leave it as an open question whether a machine whose body is just like a human's but whose insides may or may not be similar to ours could think like us.

Otto's workbook: Let's continue the thought experiment we just left off but take it in a slightly different direction. Imagine you're walking to the library, chatting pleasantly with a classmate, and you think to yourself, "What a fine human to talk to." This classmate trips over a crack in the sidewalk—oh no! But when the classmate hits the sidewalk, you see their hand snap off and wires protruding from their wrist. It turns out that their insides are wires and silicon chips! Is your belief that your classmate is human a true belief?

The more you know (mini version): This is a version of the "Twin Earth" thought experiments developed by Hilary Putnam, which started debates over **content internalism** and **content externalism** in philosophy of mind. You can learn more about this in "Externalism About the Mind" and "Narrow Content" in the *Stanford Encyclopedia of Philosophy*.

8.6 Brief replies to the "too radical" and "not radical enough" worries

For the "too radical" objection, the weak embodiment theorist could just shake it off. "Oh, I'm too radical for you?" they could say, "that's fine. Let me get out the world's smallest violin to play a sad song about it." And they could even do this in a principled way! Psychology is about human behavior. Working with machines is helpful insofar as it tells us something interesting about the nature of human minds and behaviors. As soon as machines aren't helpful anymore, we don't use them. Either way, there's no reason to be concerned with whether or not machines can think as we do.

For the "not radical enough" objection, Fred Adams has a thorough reply in his chapter "Rehashing Embodied Cognition and the Neural Reuse Hypothesis" from *Current Controversies in Philosophy of Cognitive Science*. Adams notes that there is a "strong" reading of the neural reuse hypothesis and a "weak" reading. The strong reading is what we see in §8.3: the parts of the brain that are associated with motor movement also contribute to "higher" cognitive tasks; therefore, "higher" cognition is *constituted* in part by motor functions. The weak reading takes the same observations about neural activity and concludes that "higher" cognition is caused, in part, by motor functions. Adams argues that the weaker reading is consistent with both the data on neural reuse *and* weak embodied cognition.

8.7 Conclusions

So what are we left with? You might find it unsatisfying, but we've got some strong reasons for and against weak embodied cognition. If you want our advice—and it's been known to happen—weak embodied cognition is helpful to test your commitments to the disembodied mind. As you're developing your own views on the nature of the mind, ask yourself: is disembodiment enough and weak embodiment a passing fad? If there's something right about embodied cognition, does weak embodiment incorporate the body enough? Is weak embodied cognition still too weak? If you answered "no, no, yes," then you're in luck: in the next chapter, we dive into strong embodiment.

Notes

1 Now "soul" means something different for Aquinas than how we usually think of it. "Soul" comes to us from the Greek term *psuche* and the Latin term *anima*. The soul is that part of us that animates us. One contemporary reading from Bill Jaworski in his *Structure and the Metaphysics of Mind*: "soul" is a term referring to the structure of one's body and one's life. It's not a *thing* but rather a principle of organization.
2 The philosopher **Ludwig Wittgenstein** uses a similar analogy in *Philosophical Investigations* §360-361: "The chair is thinking to itself... WHERE? In one of its parts? Or outside its body; in the air around it? Or not *anywhere* at all?".
3 One of us might be writing this during a heat wave.
4 Note the "if" at the start of that sentence. You might reasonably be skeptical of the argument.
5 We're indebted to Julian Kiverstein's chapter "Embodied Cognition and the Neural Reuse Hypothesis" in *Current Controversies in the Philosophy of Cognitive Science*.
6 For details, see "Multiple Realizability" in the *Stanford Encyclopedia of Philosophy*: https://plato.stanford.edu/entries/multiple-realizability/
7 Actually, this argument was first developed as an objection to **physicalism**, which is the view that everything is physical and therefore that the mind is a physical object. But any functionalist who is also committed to functional states being realized in *some* material substance will face this objection.

9

STRONG EMBODIMENT

9.1 Chapter overview

Strong embodied cognition rethinks what cognition looks like. It gets rid of mental representations and other internal entities. As a result, it locates information for cognition in the world around us. We are sensitive and respond to that externally located information as part of thinking and acting. As a result, the divisions between perception, cognition, and action become fuzzy.

9.2 Connecting to the jazz standard

In Chapters 4 and 5, we introduced extended mind theory and some developments. In Chapter 7, we connected it with weak embodied cognition. In this chapter, we'll introduce strong embodiment. You'll notice something different about how the extended mind fits with strong embodiment. For strong embodiment, the world around the agent is built into our concept of the mind. So while extended mind theory is an add-on for weak embodiment, it's part and parcel of strong embodiment.

9.3 Introducing strong embodiment

Imagine all the things you do with a computer, laptop, or smartphone: type documents, navigate the world, text, and watch hilarious cat videos. Each one of those is enabled by an application or bit of software. If you take away the application, you can't do the thing—you can't listen to music on

DOI: 10.4324/9781003356622-11

your phone if you don't have an app for playing music; you can't take pictures without an app for taking pictures. Now, for each one of those activities—listening to music, taking pictures, watching cat videos—imagine the app were to be removed from your device. What could you do? Not a whole lot. You'd have an operating system, like Windows or MacOS or ChromeOS or Linux (nerd), but it wouldn't really have anything to operate on. Now imagine you chuck the operating system—the very thing that runs your computer. What's left now? I'm sure the computer science majors could give us some details and uses, but for most of us, we have a paperweight.

This is what's so hard about wrapping our minds around strong embodiment for the first time. We're so used to thinking about ourselves as being like computers that it's a challenge to imagine what the mind might be like if we're *not* computers.[1] We're effectively asking, "what is a computer without any software?" As a Zen kōan: what is a computer if it cannot compute? Here are a few strategies for moving from a representational view of mind to a strongly embodied view.

9.3.1 Stop thinking about minds as things people have

We often think about the mind or mental states as *things*.[2] Once we start thinking about them as things, then the next obvious questions are: how does the thing work? How is it connected to the brain? Do other animals have the thing? Could a machine have the thing? So your first step is to stop thinking about the mind as a thing. It isn't a *thing* at all![3]

This is surprisingly hard to do. In Western culture, we're surrounded by messaging and cultural artifacts that encourage us to think about the mind as a thing. Lakoff and Johnson, whom we met in Section 7.4.2.1, argue that a predominant metaphor for the mind in American English is MIND IS A CONTAINER. Notice how we talk about minds: keep something in mind, ideas floating around in the mind, putting a thought in someone's head. Lakoff and Johnson take this as evidence that not only do we tend to think about minds as things, we often think of them as containers.

Now, instead of asking what the mind is, we'll ask a different question: what do mind-terms refer to?[4] So when you say, "Ella believes that it snowed yesterday," what does the word "believe" refer to?

9.3.2 Reframe what mental terms point to

Instead of thinking about "mind" and other mental terms, like "believe" or "want," as pointing to something spatially inside of a person, think about these terms as applying to living organisms in their environments.

Some examples might help. **Aristotle** believed that character traits are revealed through many interactions. Just as one swallow doesn't make a summer (as he says in *Nicomachean Ethics*), one day of happiness doesn't make somebody a happy person. In the same way, we don't have to think about beliefs or desires as internal states. We can instead imagine them as states and actions of organisms in their environments. In this case, we could say of Babe Ruth that he believed he was playing baseball because he was doing the sorts of things that someone playing baseball does: talking strategy, swinging a bat, yelling at umpires, and so on.

In other words, when we're thinking about minds, what we actually want to focus on are activities of organism-environment systems. That's our starting point. If we're interested in thinking about how people reason, then we're better off regarding the activity of reasoning in terms of the whole organism in its environment. When we do this, we're looking not only at what's happening in the head but also at the world around the organism.

9.3.3 Find new go-to examples of thinking

When you try to imagine someone thinking, what do you picture? Is it something like Rodin's *The Thinker*: someone, deep in thought, with their chin resting on their fist? Or maybe you imagine someone sitting at their desk, their head resting in their hands, contemplating life's mysteries. In each of these examples, we have someone doing something that looks to be completely inside the head. The thinking in these cases seems to be in the head, so all thinking must be in the head.

But from the viewpoint of strong embodiment, these are not representative of problem solving. Imagine trying to make a meal with the limited ingredients of your kitchen or finding where a leak is coming from in your roof or seeing if you're free a week and a half from today at 6:30 pm or how many credits you need to graduate or preparing someone's coffee order. These are all sophisticated activities requiring a lot of cognitive horsepower. Thinking and cognition in general aren't limited to math or literature or philosophy. We problem-solve *all the time!*

> **Otto's workbook**: Describe a problem you've solved (or tried to solve) in the last week. What did you do to solve that problem (or try to solve it)?

During the writing of this book, I (CL) had a leak in my basement. I went downstairs at 5:30 am and saw two inches of water on my basement floor. After the panic subsided, I realized the first task was to stop the water from running, so I shut the main water valve (conveniently located in the basement—something I remember from having shut off the water to replace a toilet some years ago).[5] I looked around at the walls and ceiling, and there was no sign of leakage, so I inferred that it was unlikely to be a pipe inside the house. Then, I noticed that there were water stains on an exterior wall, below a small window with a lot of standing water in the window-well; I suspected there was a leak from the outside spigot and water was coming in through the window. I knew it was highly unlikely that there was a leak in the outside part of the pipe, and there was no sign of a leak on the inside stretch of pipe. I went outside to inspect. I noticed that the outdoor spigot was on, but the hose was turned off. I saw that there was a crack in part of the hose that was very close to the house and it was wet. So what happened? The hose was filled with water for quite some time (I have no idea how long). The cold weather probably rendered the old hose more brittle and maybe some of the water further down the hose had frozen, creating lots of pressure on that weak spot. At some point, the hose broke down and water began pouring out of the leak, into the window-well, and ultimately into my basement.

Why go into such detail with this mundane story? It's because the details make it clear that there was no problem-solving "in the head," even though there is plenty of cognitive work going on. Of course, I used my perceptual and motor abilities: I had to look and move around in order to find the issue. I also used what I knew to rule out possibilities. There's no easy way to do this "in the head." In fact, it's hard to imagine what doing all this "in the head" would look like. In some important ways, I needed to be in that space and free to move about as I'm solving this mystery. The roles of the environment and my body are crucial as I'm problem-solving.

Now reflect on your own experiences when you had a problem to solve. You might notice that so much of what we do in a day is this kind of problem solving! Figuring out what to make for dinner with a bottle of mustard, three slices of cheese, and some pickles is a problem that needs solving no less than calculating integrals.

But wait, there's more! Consider a wide range of flexible, adaptive behaviors: cooking, music, and sports, for instance. Each of these involves a kind of expertise of one degree or another. Cooking is a highly skilled activity and the cook has to be flexible enough to change on the fly in case they don't have the right ingredients or the flame is set too high. These are all intelligent behaviors; they require mastery to perform competently. They require a high degree of coupling with the environment that demands fast adaptation to changing conditions. Surely, these are examples of intelligent behaviors if anything is! Agents in these cases are engaged in embodied and situated problem-solving. We'll actually consider these examples of expertise in greater detail in Section 12.9.

Having this kind of stock of go-to examples for cognition is important because they make the embodied and situated nature of cognition obvious, a lot more so than other examples of cognition and intelligence. One popular test for intelligence, which conceptualizes thinking as happening in the head, is the Progressive Raven Matrices. Here's a particularly challenging one.[6] Here is the pattern (Figure 9.1).

Look carefully at the boxes. There's a pattern at work here. Now, which of the following is the most appropriate image to put in place of the dash? (Figure 9.2)

Did you figure it out? If you didn't, don't sweat it—we didn't either. First, consider the squares in the original problem going in order from the top left corner to the bottom right. In fact, let's tag these squares as A, B, C, D, E, F, G, and H. Look at where the lines end on the right side in square A and where they start on the left side of square B. The lines in square B start where the lines in square A end. The lines in square C start where the lines in square B end. The lines in square D start where the lines in square C end. Looking at the boxes this way, the only one of the choices where the lines pick up where the lines in square H end is number 5.

So why bother introducing this puzzle? It's taken as a measure of intelligence because it requires a lot of demanding abstract thinking. But—and this is the point—we rarely, if ever, engage in this kind of problem-solving. If we *do* take it as the prime example of problem-solving, then we're using

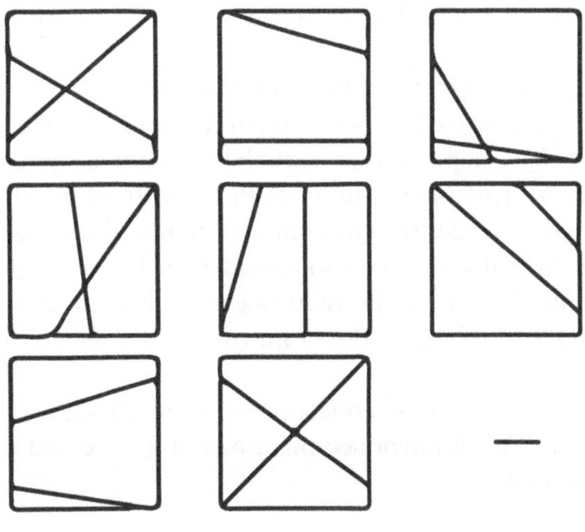

FIGURE 9.1 A challenging Raven Matrix.

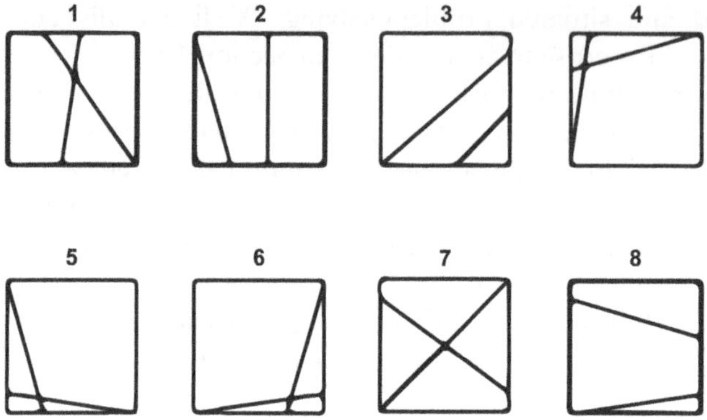

FIGURE 9.2 Possible answers for Raven Matrix.

a very rare case to define what's run-of-the-mill. That's like a straight-A student taking the one D she got on a test as representative of her academic performance.

The take-home message is that if you want to understand thinking and mental life generally, go with ordinary examples of people solving problems in their natural environments. The go-to examples of thinking for strong embodiment will involve some kind of activity. When strong embodiment folks think about thinking, they go with something less cerebral, like preparing a meal or repairing a car. There's a good reason for this. Strong embodiment, as you've guessed, is all about the body. So they choose examples of complex activities that require thinking or reflection. These kinds of examples play up how the body is a part of the cognitive system.

"But guys," we can (maybe) hear you thinking, "everything you're talking about can be described by brain activity! The environment is just inputs to that system." We suppose that could be true, but ask yourself this: what do you get out of treating the brain as the central information-processor? You still have to consider the environment: that's where the information is coming from. You also still have to consider the body. So given that, what kind of benefits do you get by reducing everything to the brain? If anything, reducing everything to the brain can encourage you to miss what's right in front of you.

We'll need a new set of concepts to begin thinking about strongly embodied minds. We'll introduce them one at a time and then pull them together at the end.[7]

9.4 A useful distinction

Edmund Husserl distinguishes between two ways of thinking about the body and its relationship to thought. The first is **Körper**, which is German for *body*. This is thinking about the body from a third-person perspective, which is what we find in the sciences. Here, we don't focus on the body from our own perspective. Instead, the sciences tell us about our bodies and how they are relevant to thinking.

The other is **Leib**. This is typically translated as the *lived body*. The literal translation is along the lines of *darling* or *dear* (as a term of affection). The idea is that we think about our bodies more intimately in characterizing our experience. *Leib*, then, is the body as it plays a role in our subjective experience. It's not just about measurable variables like heart rate but rather about how one's body affects one's experience from one's own point of view.

Here's a rough analogy with exercise. *Körper* is like having a smartwatch or smartphone that tracks facts about your body: your pulse, blood pressure, breathing rate, etc. You can track your effort by means of these measures. If your heart rate is above 140 beats per minute, then you're working hard. *Leib*, by contrast, is closer to the rate of perceived exertion. When you're exercising, you might ask yourself how long you could keep up what you're doing or how many more reps you could do. You're reflecting on your bodily state and what you think you could do.

Weak embodiment usually thinks about the body as *Körper*. We investigate the role of the body in cognition by means of third-personal, scientific research and not relying on the first-person perspective in any way. The machinery to include the role of the body in cognition is outside your awareness. It happens in neurons and the structures of representations. The role of the body in cognition couldn't *possibly* be available in consciousness. Strong embodiment usually thinks about the body as *Leib*.

9.5 Explanatory concepts

Let's get into the kind of mindset we need. When we're thinking about action, we begin with the whole animal in its environment. Suppose we see a dog chasing a squirrel. To begin understanding this behavior, we consider the dog in its environment—let's say it's running around a park. The dog sees the squirrel and it darts off after it. This is our starting point: the dog in the park chasing the squirrel. We're not worried with brains just yet; that's part of the story but just a part. The questions we ask will have to do with the whole enchilada: the organism in its environment. Some questions that come to mind might be:

1 How does the squirrel show up to the dog? As a playmate or as lunch?
2 The dog moves very quickly to catch the squirrel—how does it track the squirrel as a fast-moving object in the environment?
3 Would the dog chase another squirrel if one should happen to cross its path?
4 How does a dog move so skillfully to track the squirrel and yet not run into any trees?

Notice that, for all these questions, there will be elements of the brain involved, but we don't start our investigation at the level of the brain. We start at the level of the organism in its environment.

Otto's workbook: Use a search engine or AI to find information about beavers building dams. Why do they do it? What advantages does the behavior bring? Is it possible to explain dam-building without consideration of the environment? What would such an explanation look like? What would it be missing?

We're going to go through seven important concepts and explain how they help us understand the mind as deeply embodied: timescales, affordances, information, *Umwelt* (aka the world as the living organism experiences it), emotions, intentionality, and sense-making. What we're trying to do in the following subsections is describe some concepts that we can use to understand *Leib*, our bodily experiences from the first-person perspective.

9.5.1 Timescales

One critique of representationalism that we didn't mention before is that it doesn't take time into account as relevant for understanding cognition. This is understandable in a way. Computers work *amazingly* fast. Here's a comparison. Our brains work on the order of milliseconds—that is, thousandths of a second. For instance, it takes 3–4 ms for the sodium-ion channels in a neuron to "reset." This is fast. A computer can execute a single machine instruction in a nanosecond—that is, a *billionth* of a second. The unit for measuring neural activity is 10^3 times bigger than the unit for measuring computer activity! So, in thinking about the mind as a kind of computer, it's easy to neglect the dimension of time because computers are so fast.

However, computers aren't a good model for understanding the mind *because* they're so fast. Consider chess grandmaster Gary Kasparov playing the machine Deep Blue. Deep Blue could "see" deeper into games than

Kasparov because it was comparing 200 million positions each *second* (Greenemeier 2017). Our brains are sedated turtles compared to computers. But that's okay. The issue, then, is that because computers work so quickly, it's easy to forget that their processes unfold in time too.[8] Computers, then, aren't a good model for understanding the mind.

Where this leaves us is thinking about the relevance of time for an understanding of the mind. Often, philosophers and cognitive scientists will talk about timescales. Consider a complex phenomenon like speaking a language. If we're inquiring into processes that are involved with speaking a language, there are many "levels" we can think about. Here are some examples:

Field	*Description*	*Relevant time units*
Neurolinguistics	Investigating the role of the brain and neurons in language production and comprehension	Milliseconds
Psycholinguistics	The role of computational and/or dynamic mechanisms in language production and comprehension	Milliseconds, seconds
Developmental linguistics	How children learn a language	Days, weeks, months, years
Discourse analysis	How conversation unfolds among pairs of speakers	Seconds, minutes
Dialectology	Study of regional variations in vocabulary, grammar, and meaning	Weeks, months, years
Politeness theory	Study of ways in which people are polite and demonstrate respect to others	Days, months, years, decades
Historical linguistics	Changes in languages over various stretches in history (e.g., 1200–1500 CE)	Decades, centuries, millennia

So what is the "right" timescale for studying language? That's kind of a nonsense question. There is no "right" timescale because language is a phenomenon that crosses many timescales.

"But," you might insist, "if we're interested in how a particular person communicates, which timescale is the best?" This seems like a reasonable question, but it's motivated by the same kind of question as finding the "right" timescale. For instance, in the USA, people use "pop" and "soda" to refer to soft drinks like Coca-Cola and Pepsi. So if Jamie says, "can you get me a pop?", we might look at what's going on in the brain (neurolinguistics), why "pop" is used instead of "soda" (dialectology), or why the request is phrased in that particular way (politeness theory). Each of these has something to contribute to our understanding of Jamie's utterance.

Not only does understanding complex phenomena require looking at contributors at different timescales, but it also encourages us to think about mental phenomena as taking place over time. In any thought process, you could identify a beginning, middle, and end. This enables you to think about how that process unfolded over time.[9] For example, have you ever started a sentence and it "got away from you," so that it didn't end up where you thought it would? Or have you ever told a story that just kind of petered out? Thinking about those events as taking place over periods of time—unfolding within a specified time span—gives us new insight into the nature of those processes.

There is a field of study relevant to looking at how systems change over time: **dynamic systems theory**, which requires a lot of calculus.[10] The piece that's relevant for us is that systems are **dynamic**; they change over time. And not only do they change over time, but what happened earlier affects what happens later. Consider, for example, a hot cup of coffee on a cold winter morning. The coffee cools off faster when there's a bigger difference between the coffee's temperature and the air temperature. As the coffee's temperature drops, the rate of cooling slows down. Cooling is dynamic in the sense that future states of cooling depend on past states of cooling.

> **The more you know**: This is Newton's law of cooling: the rate at which an object cools is proportional to the difference between the object and the external temperature. It is not about how reading philosophy makes one cooler and/or more hip.

So, as we continue thinking about strongly embodied cognition, begin thinking about how thinking and other mental activities unfold over time—that is, how what came before affects what is happening now and what will happen in the future.

Philosophers like **William James** and Edmund Husserl describe our experience of time as the future bleeding into the present moment and then fading into the past. Husserl gives us the terms **protension** and **retention.** We exist in an ever-present now,[11] but how we experience the now is informed by what we expect will happen: this is protension. Our current experience is likewise informed by what has just happened: this is retention. James describes this as a kind of swelling of the future into the present and shrinking into the past.[12] And so we not only have different timescales for thinking about complex phenomena, but we also have our subjective experience of the flow of time as an aspect of our strong embodiment.

9.5.2 Affordances

Let's start with some observations. Chairs can be sat on, floors can be walked on, mugs can be picked up, stairs can be climbed, puddles can be jumped over (and in), baseballs can be thrown, and doors can be walked through.

> **Otto's workbook**: Come up with seven more examples like the ones above. Was it easy or hard? Hold on to these; we'll be coming back to them.

These properties of objects are called **affordances**. They are opportunities for action. They *afford* actions. What can you do with a chair? You can sit on it. What can you do with a mug? You can pick it up.

Affordances were introduced by **James Gibson**, and they form part of the foundations for ecological psychology. The core idea is that things in the world enable living organisms to do things, but not just any old thing. You can't drive a car with a chair and you can't walk through a wall (unless you're the Kool-Aid Man, obviously). Objects in the world provide us with specific opportunities for action. We're going to use the verb "afford" to indicate this. Chairs *afford* sitting, baseballs *afford* throwing. Additionally, we'll often say that people "pick up" or "pick up on" affordances. This is meant in a colloquial way, like when you're picking up on a hint of sarcasm in someone's tone, or when elder millennials say, "I'm picking up what you're putting down." When we need to be careful about our words, we'll talk about "perceiving" affordances.

Affordances are out there in the world to be picked up. They don't depend on us for their existence.[13] Stairs can be climbed and baseballs thrown even if there's no one around to climb or throw them. But not just any organism can pick up on any affordance. Some affordances are available to people that aren't available to mice: *you* can walk up a flight of stairs, but a mouse can't. Some affordances are available to non-human animals that aren't available to people: a mouse can squeeze underneath a closed door, but you can't.

But even within a species, not all affordances are available to everyone. Someone in a wheelchair isn't able to climb stairs and not everyone can climb a rope.[14] Affordances can also be specific to social settings and culture. In some Jewish traditions, someone observing *shomer negiah* refrains from shaking hands with members of the opposite sex.[15] Among Roman Catholics, everyone—including minors—drinking wine from the same chalice is part of celebrating the Mass. Usually, we don't see a cup touched by hundreds of mouths as affording drinking from. These are sometimes called **social affordances.**[16] We see opportunities for action in the social environment as much as the physical environment.

Affordances are likewise related to our observation that cognition happens in time. Perceptions of affordance are both affected *by* time and unfold *in* time. Different affordances are available to us at different ages and stages. A can of beer might not afford drinking when you're 18 months, but it does afford drinking when you're middle-aged. And our perception of the world takes place in time: watching a person walk by has a beginning, middle, and end. The affordance pick-up at the beginning affects what happens in the middle and subsequently the end. If it's your significant other walking by, you can afford to approach them, and those affordances available to act on change as you continue to approach them.

The shift in thinking about perception as perception of affordances means letting go of a "photographic" idea of perception, where perception is basically the eyes and brain taking snapshots of the world. Instead, we see the world in terms of what we can do; our experience of the world is of ways we can act in the world. Perception of a mug isn't about getting an accurate mental picture of a mug; it's about seeing what can be done with a mug.

Otto's workbook: What if you're not sure what can be done with an object? Write a few sentences about how you might learn more about a foreign object. How does that relate to our concept of affordances?

We'll develop this idea some more in Section 9.5.4, but affordances highlight something interesting about organisms and their environments: they are *mutually specifying*. The affordances an organism picks up on specify the environment for that organism. Similarly, the affordances in the environment specify what kinds of organisms can pick up on them. Think of it kind of like a lock and key: the shape of the key tells you what kind of lock it will open, and the structure of the lock tells you what kind of key opens it. The fact that a mouse sees the gap under a door as passable says something about the mouse's relationship to its environment as well as the environment's relation to the mouse. It's a little bit like when Goldilocks is snooping through the home of the three bears: she can tell that there is a big, medium, and small bear living there because of the sizes of their beds; their bed sizes tell her something about the bears. And looking at the bears would tell her something about what size beds they need.

9.5.3 Information in the environment and sensorimotor enactivism

What is **direct perception**? Organisms have direct contact with the world. When I touch the table, my experience is of my hand touching the table. There's no internal representation mediating the experience—if there were, that would count as **indirect perception**. (Bertrand Russell once commented that the only thing we really see is the back of the retina.[17]) So what is perception then if it's not an internal picture of the external world? We'll talk about this a little bit later, but the key idea is that perception is reimagined in a way that involves a kind of "openness" to the world around us. Another way of thinking about it is that the world is "given" to us in perception. It is you yourself, and not some subpart of you, that perceives. The organism does the perceiving: *you* perceive, not your eyes, ears, or brain. Eyes, ears, and brains (among other things) are part of perceiving, but they don't do the perceiving.

Sensorimotor enactivism is a theory about action and direct perception. Developed in detail by Alva Noë (among others), sensorimotor enactivism holds that perception is a whole-body enterprise. We'll introduce more examples in Section 9.5.3.2, but just notice a few things. Our eyes are constantly moving (i.e., saccading), and we move our bodies in order to have a look at things. The environment shows up for us in predictable ways during perception. Just notice that when you walk toward a tree, it takes up more room in your visual field. That's all to say, perception is done by people, not brains. And we learn how to see by moving around the world. So we don't need internal representations when perception and perceptual experience are understood as active, as things we do rather than as something that happens to us.

9.5.3.1 Information in the environment

If meaning is in the world around us, then strong embodiment theorists who are interested in explaining human behavior need some kind of story for how meaning outside us shapes behavior *without* appealing to internal representations.

Let's get into this by way of an analogy. Imagine a sidewalk or trail for a moment.

> **Otto's workbook**: Go on and draw a sidewalk or trail leading *away* from you.

You'll notice that the outside edges of the sidewalk or trail get closer as they move into the distance. You can notice this if you're ever standing on railroad tracks. As the rails move away from you, they vanish into a point far in the distance.

This is a constant in our perception of the world. Distance affects how things show up for us. Things further away look smaller than things closeup; parallel lines converge in the distance. In the 15th century, Italian artist and architect Filippo Brunelleschi was among the first in Western art to incorporate perspective. Part of the genius of Leonardo da Vinci's *Mona Lisa* is his use of perspective: he includes atmospheric perspective. The color of the sky lightens as it moves toward the horizon, which is just the effect of the atmosphere on our perception.

Gibson's key insight was that these perceptual regularities are not distortions or tricks of the mind—they are sources of information about the world. As we move, the entire visual field shifts in structured ways. This structured change is called **optic flow**: the systematic transformation of visual information that occurs as an organism moves through its environment. Optic flow is not something constructed internally; it is lawfully generated by the relation between organism and world. Because of this, movement reveals information already available in the environment.

For example, imagine you're a pilot trying to land your plane on a runway. As you descend, the visual scene expands outward from a central point, and the edges of the runway shift in predictable ways. If we wanted to represent this in an illustration, it might look something like this (Figure 9.3).

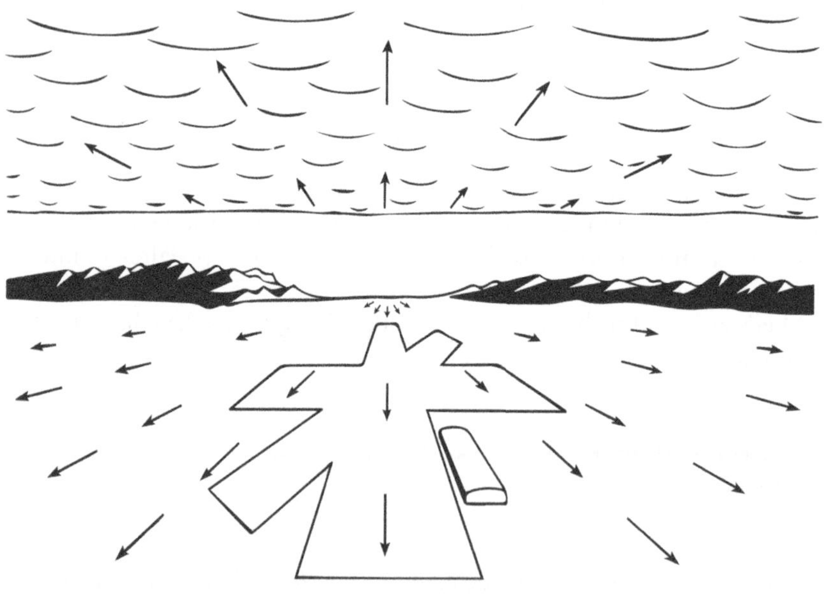

FIGURE 9.3 Optic flow during forward motion toward a runway. As an observer moves forward and downward, visual features expand outward from a central point on the horizon (the focus of expansion), providing information about direction and motion relative to the environment.

The arrows indicate the direction of the optic flow. As you fly forward and downward, the scenery expands outward from a central point and streams past you. Looking at the image, you can even feel a faint sense of forward motion toward the horizon. Artists use this trick all the time. If you're a fan of comic books or graphic novels, you'll see lines like these to indicate movement or action, especially if the action is meant to feel perspectival and immersive.

What we're doing is describing the environment as it appears to a situated perceiver. Doing this can take some getting used to. Imagine you're sitting at a circular table. What shape does it appear to be from where you are? It does not appear perfectly circular. It would look circular only from directly above. Seated at the table, it appears elliptical. And suppose there's some light coming from a lamp in the corner: does it appear as though the table is evenly illuminated? No—the side closer to the light appears brighter than the side farther away.

This is a shift in our mindset: we're not describing things from a detached, God's-eye perspective. Instead, we're beginning with how the world shows up for a perceiver at a particular place and time. The reason this is so fruitful (and merely subjective) is that our perceptual systems and their interactions with the world exhibit lawful regularities across perceivers. If someone stood on the railroad tracks and, looking as they go off into the distance, said "no, it doesn't appear to me like those rails converge towards a point on the horizon," you would reasonably suspect confusion or dishonesty. The convergence is not a private illusion; it is a lawful feature of how the world appears to embodied perceivers moving within it.

9.5.3.2 Sensorimotor enactivism

Remember our mention of sensorimotor enactivism a few paragraphs ago? The core idea is that perception is **enacted**. We enact perception through our embodied engagement with the world. You learn, for example, that turning your head to the left brings things on the left-hand side of your peripheral vision more fully into view. And when we say you "learn" this, we mean it in the way that you learn how to ride a bike. It isn't taught to you by means of propositions; it's a coordinated pattern of bodily movement and perceptual change that becomes second nature. These are *sensorimotor contingences* that structure perception. Our perceptual lives unfold in accordance with these contingencies.

Here's another example. When you hear something faint, you'll often turn an ear in the direction of the noise. This makes sense: orienting your head changes the acoustic information available to you. Is hearing merely the reception of soundwaves entering the ear canal and triggering a biological chain of events? For the sensorimotor enactivist, the movement of the head (and body) is constitutive of the act of hearing.

Consider your favorite food or drink. Imagine how you experience those flavors in your mouth: if you love chocolate ice cream, you might move it across your tongue this way and that to better enjoy the flavor. Or if you're a beer or whiskey connoisseur, you might hold the alcohol in your mouth to linger on particular flavors—very differently than if you were swallowing cough medicine as quickly as possible. In fact, compare the way you drink your favorite beverage to any kind of gross, medicinal syrup. It's unlikely that you drink the syrup in the same way you drink the beverage. In both cases, you're drinking something and tasting it, yet your bodily engagement shapes the experience itself. You're doing something to savor or avoid those flavors.

For sensorimotor enactivism, perception is active, not passive. IIt is something whole organisms do, not something performed by isolated neural subsystems. But why think about perception in this way?

First, it resonates with our lived experiences. Consider that you're holding this book (or e-reader). Pause and notice your bodily state. Are your hands and arms tired from holding the book? What about your neck—are you tilting your head down, up, or looking at the book straight ahead? How close does the book need to be to your face for you to see the letters clearly? How tightly are you holding the book? Each of these factors shapes your perceptual experience. If your neck is tired or hurting, you might have a harder time focusing on the letters. The same goes for your arms. If the letters are looking blurry, you'll bring the book closer to your face. If your eyes are strained by glare, you'll pull the book back. We do all of these things without thinking about it—it's automagic.[18] From this perspective, it would be strange *not* to take the body into account. Our bodies aren't just for hauling the perceptual equipment around. Our bodies are themselves part of the perceptual system.

Second, it aligns with findings from neuroscience. Recall Michael Anderson's findings from §7.3.2.2 The key idea is that lots of parts of the brain are involved in all kinds of tasks; it's unlikely that there are perception- or language- or or other neatly isolated centers. Part of the lesson is that neural structures involved in perception and action are activated in overlapping sets of tasks. Given this fact about neural organization, we can compare two theories: one in which action and perception are distinct activities or one in which they are deeply integrated. Of the two, the second better fits the organization of neural structures. This approach offers a scientifically grounded account of perception that bridges the gap between the mechanics of sensory systems (e.g., blind spots, saccades) and the richness of lived experience (e.g., the seamless visual field we actually experience).

9.5.3.3 The environment moves you

You may have had this experience. In the Seattle–Tacoma International Airport (and many others), there are relatively narrow corridors leading to gates for flights. Sometimes there are stores you can pop into; they're typically "convenience" stores or shops for picking up a last-minute item before boarding. In the corridors, the environment invites you to keep moving. The space is designed to encourage forward movement. Sure, you could stop if you wanted to, but you risk disrupting the flow of foot traffic. In Gibsonian terms, these architectural features structure different fields of affordances: narrow corridors afford transit; open plazas afford dwelling.

But these corridors are interrupted by large spaces with high ceilings. These larger spaces typically have restaurants or cafés and tables. The sense of being propelled forward fades–or is at least significantly diminished. These spaces invite you to linger.

This phenomenon isn't unique to airports. Consider different kinds of public spaces. Woodland trails invite movement; open fields invite lingering. City plazas with benches afford sitting, while sidewalks encourage walking. Some spaces present mixed affordances. Some suburbs will have sidewalks, crosswalks, and bike lanes along roads with four lanes of fast-moving traffic in a single direction.

Otto's workbook: Do you ever find that you spend time in one part of your house or apartment more than others? Look around that space. Is there anything in the space that encourages you or others to stay there?

The mixed signal is that crosswalks and sidewalks afford pedestrian movement, while the speed and volume of traffic simultaneously discourage it.

The lesson? Physical spaces can be organized in ways that encourage certain kinds of behaviors, like walking or sitting. The space makes some affordances very salient and downplays others. We experience the environment as encouraging some actions and discouraging others.

9.5.3.4 Bad design

Have you ever pulled on a door that was meant to be pushed? Don't feel bad; this is often due to bad design. A handle on a door should look as if it's made to be pulled or pushed. If it's ambiguous, then it's a poorly designed handle. In other words, the affordances of that handle are not clear: the same object solicits two incompatible actions.

Side quest: The architect Katerina Kamprani has a collection of objects she designed called "The Uncomfortable."[19] They are objects that are "deliberately inconvenient." You can find them at https://www.theuncomfortable.com. Here is "The Uncomfortable Broom":

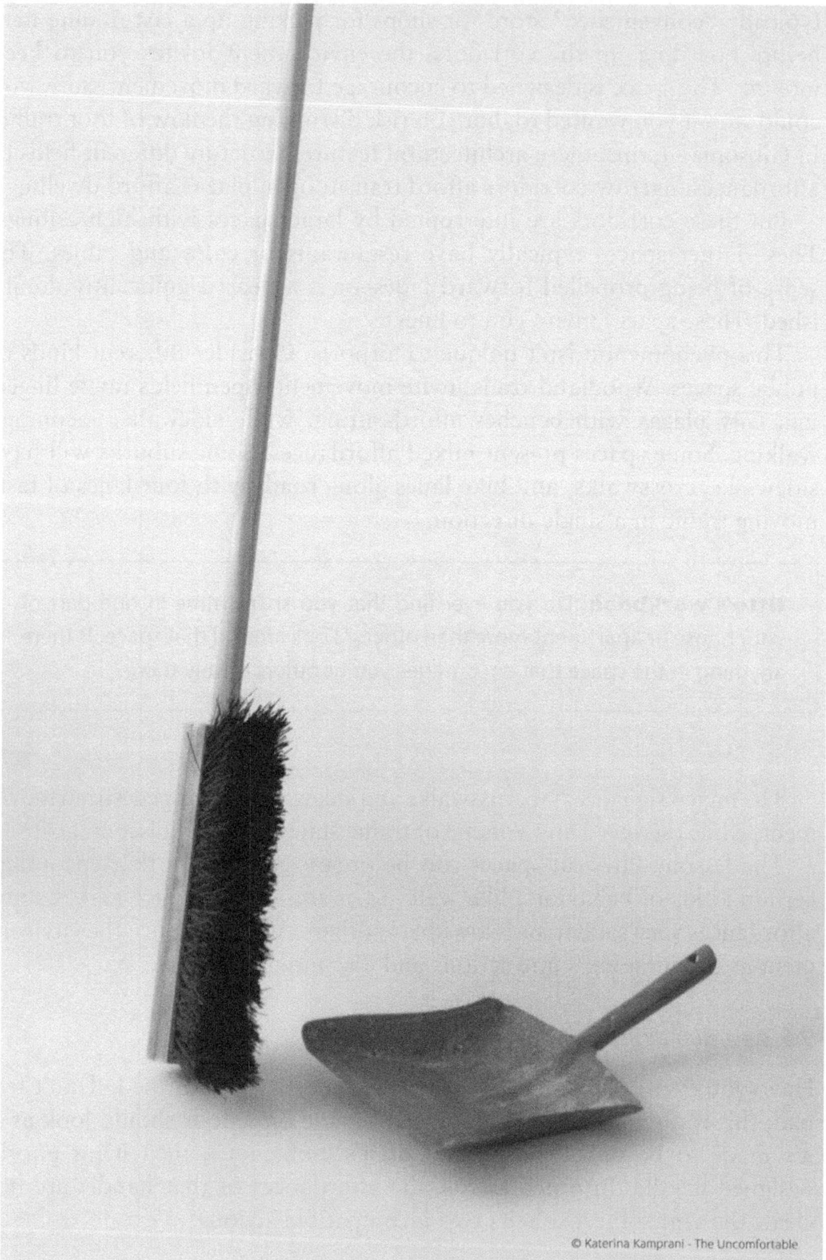

FIGURE 9.4 The uncomfortable broom.

What affordances does this broom frustrate? (Figure 9.4)

Or consider a smartphone you've just purchased. Typically, you'll find several buttons on the side: two are for volume and one is the "power" button for waking up your phone. If those three buttons are evenly spaced, then it's not obvious which is the power button and which is the volume. This problem is avoided by locating the volume buttons close to each other and the power button further away.

Instances of bad design are unclear affordances. The object is either unclear about the actions it solicits or actively nudges you in the wrong direction. The information in the environment is ambiguous.

9.5.4 Umwelt

"*Umwelt*" is a German word. The prefix "um" means (among other things) "around" and "Welt" means "world." So *Umwelt* is the world around the organism. But it's not just the world around the organism as it is described by physics or biology. Instead, it's the world around the organism as it shows up for the organism.

The more you know: So why do we use the German term "*Umwelt*" instead of translating it into English? If you translate "*Umwelt*" into English, you get "environment," which is accurate but doesn't quite capture the sense we need. "*Umwelt*" isn't just the environment; it's the environment as it is relevant and shows up for an organism. An organism's *Umwelt* is charged with meaning and value: it's not just what is out there but what is out there as it relates to me as good or bad. I (CL) am currently sitting on my couch. I see a fan nearby. I'm feeling warm, so the fan is something desirable for me—it's something that can help cool me off. It's not one thing among many in my environment—after all, there's also laundry that needs to be folded, an empty coffee mug, and a TV remote—but rather something that responds to one of my immediate interests: cooling off. So what "*Umwelt*" expresses that "environment" doesn't is the sense that the world shows up for organisms as meaningful.

Two more things: nouns in German are always capitalized, hence "*Umwelt*" instead of "*umwelt*." And the plural of "*Umwelt*" is "*Umwelten*."

Jakob von Uexküll, one of the first thinkers to use the term, encourages us to think about how the world looks for organisms given the perceptual equipment and interests of that organism. A simple example is a bacterium that consumes sugar. Its only job is to head in the direction of sugar. For that bacterium, there is only sugar and not sugar. It has no need to know about anything else; nor can it detect anything else. So if we imagine the world through the perceptual equipment of the bacterium, we'd see only sugar.

The central insight is that all living organisms have things that are and are not of relevance to them. Their worlds are made up of what is of relevance, and nothing else shows up for them.

Otto's workbook: Read up about your favorite insect: spiders, ants, crickets, lightning bugs, roly polys, whatever. Most importantly, learn about their perceptual systems and what they need to survive and reproduce. In a few paragraphs, describe the *Umwelt* of your chosen insect. A great place to start is "The Thoughts of a Spiderweb" in *Quanta Magazine*, where the author reports on (among other things) a series of studies suggesting that spiderwebs hold and process information for spiders. If you'd like to read the study that the *Quanta* essay is based on, it is "Extended spider cognition," by Hilton F. Japyassú and Kevin Laland in *Animal Cognition* 20: 2017, pp. 375–395.

We can apply this idea to humans. We occupy *Umwelten* as well. Unlike our sugar-seeking bacteria, human *Umwelten* are terribly complicated. Consider for a moment the many interests and projects you have and how they are nested in one another. Right now, you're reading a book—you're focusing on the words on the page, and what matters to you are conditions like lighting and temperature. You have many other things going on in your life, but those don't matter right now. You might need to get the oil changed in your car or you might need to pick up your niece at daycare, but you're focused on reading this book. Your *Umwelten* in the here and now consist of the book and other things in your current environment. But your *Umwelten* also consist of longer-term projects, like learning about embodied cognition.

Human *Umwelten* are layered with social and cultural features. When you walk into a classroom, there will likely be a desk and table at the front. You *could* sit there if you wanted to, but it doesn't show up for you (typically) as someplace you could sit. When you're headed for your seat on the first day of class, the desk and seat at the front of the room might as well not be there. That's because American classrooms have, as a social norm, that students don't sit at the desk and chair in the front.

Now, you might be skeptical of the notion of an *Umwelt*. After all, people's *Umwelten* will be a little different, so what generalizations could possibly be made? That's true, in a sense. For example, consider that women often have to be a lot more attuned to their surroundings late at night than men do.[20] So what shows up in a woman's *Umwelt* might be different than what shows up in a man's *Umwelt*. And you can make the same point across genders, races, and social classes. But there are two points to make here. First, there will be some things that are common across all social and cultural groups, and these will often be things that relate to our survival as organisms. A bus coming down the road in your direction is perceived as a threat irrespective of your race, gender, or social class.[21] Second, understanding experience in terms of *Umwelten* can help develop empathy and understanding, providing insights into how others live in the world. For example, African Americans sometimes see police officers as potential threats, while Caucasian Americans might not. So when asking why (for example) a Black man might run when approached by the police, we get better answers when we consider how the approaching police officer shows up for the Black man in his *Umwelt* as opposed to a White person's *Umwelt*.

9.5.5 Emotion

As mentioned in Section 7.6, emotions have a weird place in philosophy.

Side quest: Emotions have a weird place because they ride the line between mental and physical phenomena. They're mental in the sense that emotions are like thoughts in that they are about things: you can believe that *The Godfather* is a terrible movie and you can also be angry that so many people you respect like *The Godfather*. But emotions have a clear physical component as well. When you're angry, your body feels a certain way and you have specific physiological reactions. The philosopher William James had an interesting view on the relationship between thoughts and feelings. It's not that we have the mental state of an emotion and *that* causes the feeling. Instead, we have a bodily reaction and *that* causes the emotional state. Read §2 of the *Internet Encyclopedia of Philosophy* entry about William James, paying special attention to section (c): "Emotion and Will." Do you agree with James' position? Why or why not? You can learn more about James' position in §4.c of the entry "Theories of Emotion" in the *Internet Encyclopedia of Philosophy*.

For us, it's clear that emotions are involved in our mental life and also that they have a bodily component. For example, when you are angry or sad, there's a certain way your body feels. It's hard to describe exactly, but you can usually get pretty close. When you're angry, there's a kind of heat in your body. Your body tenses and your jaw clenches. You might speak more loudly, or you could be one of those creepy types who gets very quiet and steady when raging. The point is, all of our emotions, there are physical feelings that go with them that are part of what makes that emotion what it is.

There are a lot of theories about the role of emotion in our cognitive lives. We don't need to go through all of them, but there are a few points we need to get on the table. First, emotions have a **valence**: they represent the world as good or bad, worth pursuing or worth avoiding. When I am overjoyed at the birth of my first child, my feelings tag this as a good thing. When I am afraid of getting hit by a bus, my fear tags getting hit by a bus as a bad thing. It's important to note that valence isn't just about what's good or bad. It's also about what we care about. When you are angry, frustrated, and sad that you studied your hardest for an exam and still got a D, you have the emotions you have because you cared about doing well. Your anger, frustration, and sadness are a result of you caring about the exam.

Second, emotions can change the way that the world shows up for us. When you're depressed, for example, the world looks and feels different. There are different (and fewer) opportunities for action. Events that might ordinarily afford feelings of excitement or joy do not afford those kinds of responses.[22]

Third, emotions are important with respect to motivation. When we feel in danger, we are motivated to run away.[23] When you're happy, you're motivated to do a lot of different things: say "hello" cheerfully to a neighbor, whistle pleasantly, wave to acquaintances, etc. Here's a favorite story of ours. The children's book author Maurice Sendak—best known for *Where the Wild Things Are*—received a drawing from a young boy. Sendak sent the boy a note saying "thank you" and drew a Wild Thing on the back of the note. The mother wrote Sendak to report that the boy was so excited to get the drawing that he ate it. His excitement motivated him to eat the drawing.[24]

Emotions are important in a theory of embodied cognition because they bridge bodily feelings and thoughts. They're often important parts of explanations for thoughts and actions. For example, consider my (CL) flooding basement example from earlier. What might I have been feeling? At the moment, it was alarm. I let a few four-letter words fly and then focused on the task at hand—my emotional state quickly transitioned from alarm to focus. It wasn't the sort of focus you need when studying calculus; it was the kind of focus needed for accomplishing a very important task in as brief a period of time as possible. So even though I was feeling focused, the feeling of alarm hadn't quite left.

What was most salient to me in the moment was the water pouring in and the water on the floor. What I *didn't* attend to was the extension cord lying in the water. (Thank goodness there were no electricity-conducting parts in the water.) If I were feeling calm, I likely would have noticed this hazard. My alarm-tinged focus was a double-edged sword. On the one hand, it enabled me to home in on the task to be accomplished. On the other hand, I neglected situational factors that could have caused me serious harm.

My alarm and focus have felt qualities to them. When I was alarmed, my heart began to pound, the muscles in my neck and upper back tensed up, and I was speechless (minus the salty language). Focus has a feeling of a singular goal. Other thoughts drop away as I focus on the goal. In a way, even the sense of time drops away. The only thing of any value in the moment was accomplishing the task. My neck muscles were still tense, but the shift to focus brought with it the feeling of movement in my legs, arms, and torso as I moved toward the valve and pulled it closed.

We can play out how else this story might have gone. Alarm could have paralyzed me. I would have been unable to move or think. In this case, alarm would quickly shade into terror, which is characterized by thoughtlessness and lack of movement. When in a state of terror, there's little (if anything) one could do to get the agent thinking and moving again, except by shifting them from a state of terror to something else.

9.5.6 Intentionality

You were introduced to intentionality in Section 3.3.3. You'll remember that intentionality is often taken as the "mark of the mental," that is, what distinguishes mental stuff from physical stuff. When we introduced intentionality with disembodiment, we said it is a mental state's "aboutness." The belief that Frank Sinatra is from Hoboken is about *Frank Sinatra being from Hoboken*. Thoughts and language seem to have this feature of intentionality, but nothing else. This take on intentionality holds that there's a mental object that is the object of the mental state. This is a view that fits nicely with a representational view of mind.

On a strong embodied view, intentionality looks a little bit different. We're avoiding representational views in this chapter (and with strong embodiment in general). This is probably going to be the hardest of the conceptual shifts we talk about in this book, but it's important, so we'll take it slow.[25]

Let's have a belief we can keep coming back to. Suppose you glance at your desk and you believe that there is a coffee cup on the desk. There is the content of your belief that the coffee cup is on the desk. But let's look at this in a little more detail. The cup exists in time; it doesn't blip out of existence the moment you're not looking at it. In other words, it has *temporal duration*. Also, you know that cups are three-dimensional objects. While you can't see the other side of it, you have a sense of its existence. That is, the cup takes up room in space. The cup is also graspable by you.

When we're reflecting on our belief about the cup in this way, we begin with what seem to be really obvious facts about our experience—facts so obvious they hardly merit mentioning. I mean, *of course*, the cup has temporal duration. *Of course*, it has a backside even though we can't see it. But we want to pay really close attention to our experience, particularly to those things that we might take for granted.

The more you know: This approach in philosophy is called phenomenology. Its founding is most often associated with Edmund Husserl. His approach to philosophy is to begin with a "bracketing" of questions of existence and to consider what shows up for us in our experience. From there, Husserl begins thinking about the structure of experience—what has to be true of us if we're to have the kinds of experiences we have of the world.

One of the things we notice about our experience is that there's a difference between seeing a coffee cup and imagining one. After all, you wouldn't try to pour real coffee into an imaginary mug. This tells us that seeing real coffee cups and imagining coffee cups are two different kinds of experiences. They might both involve coffee cups in some way (i.e., seeing versus imagining), but they are definitely different sorts of experiences. Here's one of the big differences. When we see a coffee cup, our beliefs about the cup are about the cup itself as it exists out there in the world. When you believe that the cup is on the table, what is *not* given to you in your experience is that your belief is actually about a *representation* of the cup (as the weak embodiment theorists would say).

Otto's workbook: Imagine for a moment that your beliefs about the cup were actually about a mental representation of the cup. What would your experience have to be like for that to be true?

This is what is characteristic of intentionality on a strong embodiment view. Our beliefs, thoughts, and experiences of the world are directed toward the world itself. Husserl declared in his book *Logical Investigations* that philosophy is to go "back to the things themselves," meaning that we are to carefully consider our experience of the world exactly as we have it. When we go back to the things themselves, we're understanding ourselves as connected and involved with the world. Right now, consider that you're reading this in a book or on a screen. You adjust the book so it's comfortable in your hands and so it's easy to see the words. Maybe you're reading this on a smartphone and the phone dims the lighting on the screen for you to make it easier to read. You adjust in your seat to get a bit more comfortable. You take a sip of coffee to stay alert and momentarily take your eyes off the words—but you pick right back up again where you left off. All of your experience suggests that you're actually holding a book or reading device. Nothing in your current experience suggests that you're imagining or hallucinating a book or that the direct object of perception is anything other than this book (or whatever) you're holding. So when we think about the nature of the mind and the world, we begin with these experiences: holding a book that has sides, you can't see but know are there and that exists through time. These experiences suggest that you are engaged with the world around you. Your thoughts about coffee cups *are not* about coffee cups in the way that *Moby Dick* is about a guy with a whale obsession. Your thoughts about coffee cups are about how you are engaged with the coffee cup. Sometimes, philosophers describe this as being "geared into" the world: you are engaged with the world in the ways gears are engaged with a larger machine.

You can think about this in a *negative* way and in a *positive* way. The negative way is that intentionality, understood as part of how we *represent* the world to ourselves, is wrong. So the "aboutness" of our thoughts is not the contents of our thoughts pointing to a reality outside of the mind. You don't have an internal picture of the world that then goes on to point at something out in the world. The relationship between you and the world isn't like that of a photo to the real deal.[26] The positive way to think about it is that the "aboutness" of our thoughts is actually a kind of openness to the world. The boundary between subject and object isn't nearly as clear as a representational view of the mind suggests. We are embedded and part of the world. We're deeply connected to it.

For strong embodiment, the relationship between you and the world is more like the Doppler effect (bear with us). You know what it is even if you don't know the name. If you've ever had someone drive by you listening to music at an incredible volume, you might have noticed that the pitch changes when they get further away. That's the Doppler effect: sound waves from a moving source change relative to the location of the hearer. The result is that the pitch of the music drops the further away the car gets. (Search for "doppler effect sound example" if you want to learn more.) Ok, so here's the thing: the Doppler effect isn't something separate from the sound waves. It's a behavior of the sound waves; it's a way that the soundwaves exist. You can't separate the effect from the sound waves themselves. In the same way, you can't separate your experience of the world from the world itself. The world exists independently of your experience (just like soundwaves exist independently of the Doppler effect). But your experience of the world can't be sliced off from the world. We have experiences of the world, of each other, and of each other being in the same world; being in the world is a way that we exist. These are the building blocks of our experience of the world.

9.5.7 Sense-making

The final notion we'll introduce is that of **sense-making**. In a way, it pulls together a lot of the ideas we've seen so far.[27] Sense-making begins with an idea we've seen: that environments are meaningful for organisms, and the meaningfulness isn't imposed on the environmental stimuli but rather a product of the organism's interests in the world. These interests are shaped by our being embodied and particularly by our affective states—emotions, moods, feelings, etc. The world for organisms is *inherently* meaningful for them, and meaning is made (for them) through *action*.

To say that an organism engages in sense-*making* is to say that the organism participates in the construction of meaningfulness for itself. The states of an organism—particularly its affective states—are part of how the world shows up in meaningful ways. Sense-making is a *relational* activity; it takes place between the organism and the world. It's *through* action/activity that sense is *made*–organism and environment in interaction. We act on the world and the world "acts" right back.

Otto's workbook: A relational *property* is a property that holds of two or more entities (depending on the property). For example, "is taller than" is a relational property. It can only be true if there are two people whose heights we're comparing. Saying, "Sue is taller," without someone to be taller than is nonsense. "Is between" is also a relational property for three objects: the mug is between the lamp and the phone. A relational *activity*, then, is one in which the activity requires two or more entities. Consider "chases," as in "the dog chases the squirrel." It's nonsense to say "the dog chases." Naturally, we'd ask, "chasing what?" Come up with five examples of relational activities. Do you notice any similarities among them?

Just like chasing, sense-making is an activity that requires both the organism and the environment. The verb "sense-make" is a bit clunky, so instead we can say, "the dog makes sense of the speeding squirrel," which is a way of saying that the squirrel shows up as meaningful for the dog in a particular way.

People use "makes sense" in a colloquial way, like when someone tells you that they're going for a run to stay in shape. "Oh, that makes sense." What are some similarities and differences between this ordinary way of saying something "makes sense" and our specific usage of "making sense" (or, "sense-making")?

The connection with biology is that sense-making is a function of an organism's capacity to metabolize. Being able to metabolize means that the organism adopts a perspective of value on the world. Metabolizing organisms need food to survive; certain kinds of foods are valuable for each kind of organism (e.g., sugar for some bacteria, grass for cows, spinach for humans, etc.). So as living beings we are, by our very biological nature, sense-making.

The more you know: At the heart of one variety of strong embodiment, called **autopoietic enactivism**, is the belief that mind and life are continuous: being minded is a particular way of being a living organism. Bacteria are living organisms, just like people. But people are minded—that is, we "have" minds in a way different from bacteria. Being minded is how we are a particular biological organism. With that pillar in place, many enactivists develop concepts of cognition with biological concepts from **Humberto Maturana** and **Francisco Varela**, two theoretical biologists from the 20th century.

As another part of the concept, *affect* plays an important role in sense-making. When something is valuable or important to us, we take a specific affective stance. A growling dog is important because it could be a source of danger and we are afraid. Seeing the growling dog as a threat is for us to become afraid and make sense of the dog as a threat. These aren't two different processes: being afraid the sense-making. Being afraid is part of the sense-making. There is no sense-making without some emotion or feeling.

Finally, sense-making connects with what is *meaningful* for us. You can piece this together from the previous two paragraphs. Affect—our emotional experiences—is part of sense-making. We also have a value-driven perspective of the world in part because of our biological needs. When we make sense of the world, we perceive meaning in the world.[28] As we saw in Chapters 3 and 7, representational views assert that meaningfulness is located in minds and imposed on the world around us: the sounds we make when talking aren't meaningful in themselves. Rather, they're meaningful because we assign meaning to those noises. But when we think about how we engage the world in terms of sense-making, it's the world around us that's meaningful, and we pick up on that meaningfulness. Meaningfulness isn't entirely in the head.

9.6 Conclusion: pulling it all together

We've covered a lot of ground in this chapter. Let's see if we can pull it all together.

Our go-to example of thinking isn't the scholar sitting in their study, contemplating the mysteries of the universe. It's the tired parent who has paper napkins but not coffee filters to make their morning pot of coffee, or the mechanic figuring out why the engine is going "clunk" instead of "clang." This kind of problem solving emphasizes that the vast majority of our mental activity is bodily engagement with the world. The world doesn't supply inputs to the cognitive machinery; the world is part of the thinking activity and conscious experience. An important piece of the bodily engagement is emotion. Emotion is kind of a boundary between what's typically conceived of as physical and as mental: it has feet in both worlds. Emotion and bodily engagement with the world are a part of our sense-making activity, which is a function of our being alive and co-creating meaning in the world.

In the chapter on weak embodiment, we extended weak embodiment to include extended cognition: the view that the world outside the head is a part of the cognitive system. We can't do the same kind of thing with strong embodiment because strong embodiment by design is world-involving. As soon as you're on board with strong embodiment, you've included the wider world in the cognitive system. Just take a look at some of the key concepts: direct perception, *Umwelt*, and affordances. For instance, affordances are opportunities for action as they are presented in the environment. There's no need to extend strong embodiment; we're extended in virtue of being embodied.

There's one final point to be made that we haven't yet made explicit. Much work in Western philosophy supposes a dichotomy between mind and world. Mind is *in here* (*points to skull*) and the world is *out there* (*gestures wildly at everything*). Strong embodiment theorists, particularly Varela, Thompson, and Rosch (1991), resist that kind of dichotomy because it leads to intractable problems that the Western tradition has wrestled with literally for centuries. You could say that everything is mind-dependent (i.e., be a subjectivist, aka idealist, like **George Berkeley**) or you could say that everything is mind-independent (i.e., be an objectivist, like **Thomas Hobbes**). Strong embodiment theorists reject this dichotomy: neither subjectivism nor objectivism is right. The world is not pre-given to us as the objectivist would say; nor is the existence of the world entirely on us, as the idealist would say. Instead, our experiences of the world are of a domain that is shaped by our own activities. We navigate an ever-changing world that responds to our actions, but in a way that reveals that the world has its own rules for operating. We adapt and respond to a changing world that is itself adapting and responding to our actions. It's a constant back-and-forth of adjustments as part of making our way through the world. This is neither a mind-independent objectivism nor a mind-dependent subjectivism. It is a *middle way* (to use the lingo of Varela, Thompson, and Rosch).

Finally, you'll notice that we don't explicitly lay out arguments here as we do in other chapters you've seen so far. The reason for that is expository. Given our years of teaching and working in the tech sector, the ideas behind strong embodiment aren't as familiar as the ideas underlying disembodied views of mind. Rather than giving arguments for why strong embodiment is superior, we have instead opted to describe some central concepts. But suppose you did want to run an argument about the superiority of strong embodiment. What would that look like? You'd likely offer an **inference to the best explanation**, showing that the sorts of accounts of mind offered by a strong embodiment position are better than others on offer. Your primary source of evidence will likely be appeals to experience. Strong embodiment, drawing on phenomenological concepts, prioritizes *Leib* over *Körper*, making the case that strong embodiment views fit better with our experiences.

Of course, no view is without its concerns. We discuss some in the next chapter.

Notes

1 One of us (CL) wrote his dissertation proposal about representationalism and language. Only later was he converted to embodiment.

2 Ludwig Wittgenstein (1958, §308) has a wonderful line that's relevant here: "For we have a certain conception of what it means to learn to know a [mental] process better. (The decisive movement in the conjuring trick has been made, and it was the very one that seemed to us quite innocent.)" The "decisive movement" here is the assumption that "mind" refers to a thing—that because "mind" is a noun, it must name some entity. The conjuring trick, then, is to make it seem as though there is some inner thing—*the* mind—when what we may really have is a misleading way of speaking.

3 One of our reviewers reminds us that this is a very strong view! On its most radical reading, it rejects the idea that there are mental states or even mental imagery. So must you reject mental states in order to count as a strong embodiment theorist? No, you don't. It's possible to reject mental states in *some* domains (such as perception) while retaining them in others (like memory or imagination). We're presenting strong embodiment in its most radical form to give you a sense of just how far it can depart from traditional views. But always keep in mind that there are more moderate views on offer. Are there mental states? Perhaps—but for now, we're bracketing that question.

4 This kind of strong view has significant implications for other questions in philosophy of mind. For example, if minds are not things, what does it mean to be the same person over time? You can't simply appeal to mental states at one time and compare them to mental states at another. In fact, rejecting "thing" views of mind requires us to rephrase the question. Instead of asking whether the *same mind* persists, we may need to ask how patterns of activity, embodiment, and engagement with the world exhibit continuity over time.

5 If you're reading this and you don't know where the main water shut off valve is for your apartment or home, stop reading and find it immediately. If your apartment doesn't have its own shut-off valve, contact your building's

maintenance worker or superintendent and ask what the emergency procedure is if a pipe bursts. Future-you will be grateful.

6 https://puzzleaday.wordpress.com/2019/05/12/the-worlds-hardest-ravens-matrices/

7 We won't get into all the finer distinctions here, but we'll include footnotes for anyone who wants to dig deeper.

8 Not everyone working with computers neglects time. Programmers routinely analyze how running time scales with input size. Some programs scale linearly; others scale exponentially. Exponential growth is especially problematic, since small increases in input size can lead to dramatic increases in computation time.

9 Wittgenstein, in *Philosophical Investigations*, draws attention to the strange temporal character of mental states. Suppose you are mourning and you read something that makes you laugh aloud. In that instant, did the mourning disappear? Or consider someone you love—a parent, friend, sibling, child. Is your love present only when you are consciously thinking about it?

10 An excellent place to start is *Dynamics: The Geometry of Behavior* by Ralph Abraham and Christopher Shaw. You might also look at *A Visual Introduction to Dynamical Systems Theory for Psychology* by Ralph Abraham, Christopher Shaw, and Frederick Abraham.

11 As we exist, we're never not in the now.

12 In "The Stream of Consciousness" from *The Principles of Psychology, Vol. 1.*

13 A central debate in ecological psychology concerns whether affordances exist independently of organisms or only in relation to them. Put more technically: are affordances environmental properties, or are they relational properties between organism and environment? For a helpful overview, see Chapter 7 of Tony Chemero's *Radical Embodied Cognitive Science*. We remain neutral on this issue and will discuss affordances in whichever way best serves the exposition.

14 Just another reason why inclusive design is important.

15 There is some debate within Orthodox and Hasidic Jewish communities about how strictly this norm should be interpreted. Some maintain that any physical contact with members of the opposite sex—including handshakes—is prohibited. Others argue that a handshake as a polite social convention does not involve affectionate or lustful intent, which is the primary concern of the prohibition. See the entry on "Negiah" for an overview of the discussion: (https://en.wikipedia.org/wiki/Negiah).

16 There is ongoing debate about this issue. Some argue that whatever these phenomena are, they should not be described as *social affordances*, since "affordance" has a precise meaning in ecological psychology and extending the term risks diluting its analytical usefulness (e.g., Wilson and Golonka 2013). Others maintain that the concept of a social affordance is valuable, especially in discussions of ethnicity and social identity (e.g., Arango and Burgos 2024). Still others argue that all affordances are, in some sense, social (e.g., Baggs 2021). It is clear that the notion of social affordances remains contested.

17 I (CL) can't find the source of this quote, but it is mentioned in Ronald de Sousa's book *The Rationality of Emotions*, p. 64.

18 Automagic (*adj*): A process carried out automatically in such a clever way that the result appears to be magic. "The way the website fills in the customer information—it's automagic!"

19 Thanks to Katerina Kamprani for her permission to use this image.

20 If you're curious why, it's because women are assaulted a lot more often than men at night.

21 An exception arises in cases of severe depression and suicidal ideation. For some individuals in such states, an oncoming bus may not register simply as a threat. This illustrates how affective conditions can fundamentally alter what shows up as dangerous or valuable within one's Umwelt.
22 For discussion, see Rietveld and Kiverstein (2014).
23 Readers may be familiar with the trio of responses to danger—fight, flight, and freeze. In Chapter 15, we revisit these embodied responses in connection with mental health.
24 *The Washington Post*, "Maurice Sendak and childhood—we ate it up, we loved it," May 8, 2012.
25 Some folks might recognize that we're drawing on a lot of ideas from phenomenology to make these points about intentionality.
26 This is called "negative" because it describes what intentionality *isn't*.
27 There has been a lot of excellent work describing and expanding on the concept of sense-making. Unfortunately, we cannot cover all of it here. A great place to start is de Jaegher and di Paolo, "Participatory sense-making" (2007). For autopoietic enactivism, a strand of embodied cognition that has done a lot to develop ideas of sense-making, see *Mind in Life* (Thompson 2007) and *The Embodied Mind* (Varela, Thompson, and Rosch 2016).
28 We use "perceive" here in a literal sense. We don't do some internal calculations to ascribe meaning to events or people. We literally perceive the world in terms of meaning.

10

OBJECTIONS TO STRONG EMBODIMENT

10.1 Chapter overview

Objections to strong embodiment fall into two camps. The first comes from insiders—people who agree that there's something right about strong embodiment, but think the details still need refinement. This is what's happening when you see one strong embodiment theorist criticizing the views of another strong embodiment theorist. Since this is an intro book, we won't pursue those debates here, as they quickly get deep into the weeds. The second objection comes from critics who *aren't* sympathetic to strong embodiment and who prefer more disembodied views of mind.

10.2 Ways to raise concerns about strong embodiment

We barely scratched the surface with strong embodiment—take a look at the "Further Reading" section at the end of the book if you want more details. There are lots of internal debates, particularly about consciousness and self-awareness, but the concerns we'll raise in this chapter come from an *outsider's* perspective. In other words, we'll present a few worries voiced by those who are skeptical of the power of strong embodiment to do the kind of serious philosophical and scientific work its proponents claim it can do. In general, the kinds of criticisms we'll consider treat strong embodiment as too radical—too revisionary to count as a scientifically responsible theory of mind. So let's get right to work.

DOI: 10.4324/9781003356622-12

10.3 Conservatism in science

We introduced this briefly in Section 4.7.2. Science tends to be conservative in the sense that new discoveries build on old ones, and so scientists tend to be reluctant to discard older, foundational ideas without really good reason to do so.

Strong embodiment is radical. It requires cognitive scientists to discard representations and much of the standard internal machinery. Strong embodiment is an enormous conceptual shift: the brain is no longer the centerpiece of our mental lives. This would seem to render much of cognitive science obsolete.

As we saw in Chapter 3, the notions of representations and internal computations are *everywhere* in the sciences of the mind. More recently, **cognitive neuroscience** has made a lot of headway in identifying neural representations.[1] Given the successes of cognitive neuroscience, it's counterproductive to discard these concepts. We can put this in an argument:

1 If strong embodiment is true, then there are no neural representations;
2 If there are no neural representations, then cognitive neuroscience is fruitless;
3 Therefore, if strong embodiment is true, then cognitive neuroscience is fruitless;
4 Cognitive neuroscience is not fruitless;
5 Therefore, strong embodiment is false.

Premise 1 is a summary of some of the ideas we encountered in the last chapter. Premise 2 is another way of stating that neural representations are necessary for the success of cognitive neuroscience. Premise 3 comes from premises 1 and 2 by the rule of *hypothetical syllogism*. Premise 4 is another way of stating that cognitive neuroscience delivers a lot of empirically validated discoveries. And premise 5 comes from premises 3 and 4 by the rule of modus tollens.

There are two places where the strong embodiment theorist could push back: premises 2 and 4. Now, to apply pressure to premise 2, we have to describe how the "if" part can be true, while the "then" part is false. So how can we do this?

Recall some of the scientific concepts we introduced in the last chapter: affordances and *Umwelten*. Is it possible to develop a cognitive neuroscience of affordances? Yes! For example, Michael Anderson, has proposed a theory of neural reuse: the same neural areas can be reused in lots of different activities. One interpretation of these findings—in fact the one Anderson endorses in his book *After Phrenology*—emphasizes connections between brain, body, and world. For Anderson, affordances, and not representations, are foundational for doing neuroscience. And these are exactly the kinds of things a strong embodiment theorist can get behind.

Now, what about premise 4: cognitive neuroscience is successful. Is that true? Here's how a criticism might go. Cognitive neuroscience does not include what our mental lives are like from the first-person perspective. In fact, Thomas Nagel in his paper "What is it like to be a bat?" suggests that cognitive neuroscience could *never* give an account of our mental life from a first-person point of view. But the first-person point of view is crucial for any understanding of our mental life. Therefore, cognitive neuroscience is a failure in the sense that it will never explain all of our mental life.

Now there's another way to avoid the conclusion of the above argument: the strong embodiment theorist might reject the first premise. How? In a recent book, Shaun Gallagher (2017) suggests that strong embodiment is a philosophy of nature. It's a general orientation to ourselves and the world, but it doesn't make any scientific claims. Strong embodiment doesn't make any predictions about the effects of various interventions or describe in detail the mechanisms underpinning cognition. This move has the benefit of side-stepping objections about strong embodiment being unscientific. However, strong embodiment does in fact make claims about the nature of cognition, so it's going to have to put some skin in the scientific game at some point. This move may simply delay the inevitable confrontation with empirical questions. Sympathizers with strong embodiment will say that developing a strong scientific research agenda takes time. Critics will point out that this means the empirical facts are not yet clearly in its favor.

10.4 Scaling up

Strong embodiment is particularly powerful when it comes to perception, but it's not clear how strong embodiment can "scale up" to what is often called "higher" cognitive capacities. For example, sensorimotor contingencies explain perception in terms of gross bodily movement: moving *this* way makes the world show up like *that*. But what is it about our bodies that is involved in doing calculus, translating a book from one language to another, or balancing a budget?

Our bodies are involved in a kind of superficial way: I have to use my eyes to read and my hands to write stuff down. But the *real* cognitive work seems to be done in the head. It's really hard to see how we might provide a satisfactory account of language acquisition or learning trigonometry without appealing to internally represented information.

We saw a version of this objection in Section 3.3.1 with Noam Chomsky's critique of Skinner's behaviorist account of language acquisition. It's a kind of inference to the best explanation: given cognitivist and embodied accounts of "higher" cognition, cognitivist accounts appear to be more explanatorily powerful. Therefore, cognitivist accounts are right.

What makes cognitivist accounts more satisfactory? First, they fit with what we know about cognitive neuroscience. We can do the things we do because of the right parts of the brain doing the relevant kinds of work. And neurons either fire or do not—which is just like how information is represented in a computer. Instead of fire/not-fire, computers have 1/0. So just like a computer can do calculus in virtue of information represented in its hardware, we can do calculus in virtue of the information represented in the brain.

The more you know: Warren McCullough and Walter Pitts wrote the essay, "A Logical Calculus of the Ideas Immanent in Nervous Activity." This landmark paper made explicit how brain activity could be understood in terms of basic logic. They argued that the brain is a universal computing device.

Secondly, letting anything creep into the mechanisms of cognition that is outside the head—including the body—generates a lot of problems. Jerry Fodor (2009), in his review of Andy Clark's (2008) book on the extended mind, notes that underived content, also knows as "natural meaning" (see Section 3.5.4), is what distinguishes the mind from everything else in the world. But underived content—information that doesn't get its meaning from anywhere else—exists in the head, not in the neck or arm. It's not like losing a pinkie toe impairs your ability to do calculus.

Finally, there's so much that we do that seems to involve inference. For instance, if I see my child, her face smeared with chocolate ice cream, and I look in the trash to see the empty container of chocolate ice cream; the most obvious explanation is that my kid messily ate the ice cream. But notice something important: my conclusion—that my kid ate the ice cream—goes beyond the given facts. I see my kid covered in ice cream and an empty pint container. I have to put those two things together to come to a conclusion. It's not apparent just from looking at the scene.

The issue with inference goes even deeper; it includes any kind of **normative** judgment. If you call something stunning or hideous, brave or cowardly, reasonable or irrational, you're applying some set of criteria to the facts at hand to arrive at the conclusion. This is another case of inference. We don't see bravery or reasonableness in the way that we see a cat or a fork.

Otto's workbook: This aspect of the objection is grounded in David Hume's argument that it's impossible to get normative claims from descriptive claims. To see this, imagine a grisly scene from your favorite slasher or zombie flick. If you were to describe the scene just as you see it, you might mention blood splatters and body parts, but you would never mention that it is horrifying. Describing the scene as horrifying goes beyond what's perceivable. You have to infer that it is horrifying.

The 20th century philosopher Elizabeth Anscombe takes issue with the consequences of Hume's argument, claiming that we do see (for example) bravery. She says that bravery is a **thick concept**: a concept that has some evaluative component (e.g. good or bad) but also a descriptive component. Not just any old action counts as brave. Donating money to charity or holding the door open for the person behind you are good things to do, but they aren't brave. In 100 words, describe an instance of bravery. What do you think about Anscombe's claim that we can see bravery in the actions you describe?

It's hard to overestimate how much influence this argument has had. Andy Clark—someone who is sympathetic to embodiment—argued, along with Josefa Toribio, that there are some activities that require explanations in terms of representations. According to Clark satisfactory explanations for some human capacities, require representations. These kinds of problems are representation-hungry problems. What makes them representation-hungry is that they involve going beyond what's in front of us.

When you're planning what to make for dinner, you aren't looking at the dinner you've made. After all, you're *planning!* Explaining how we're able to do this requires entertaining states of affairs that aren't yet real. That is, we have to *represent* this future state of affairs to ourselves. Any time we are imagining, planning, or daydreaming, we're forming mental states whose contents aren't in the here and now. Those kinds of tasks seem to demand representations.

So how can the strong embodiment theorist respond? The best way is to reject the terms in which the debate is framed. Don't begin by thinking that the brain alone is where thinking happens. Don't characterize "higher" cognition in terms so abstract that the shift to information seems natural. But this move comes with a cost. There are very few points of contact between strong embodiment and cognitivism, and it's easy to see why.

One debate on which strong embodiment has weighed in a lot is theory of mind—whatever it is about us that lets us understand what other people are thinking. Two cognitivist theories are **theory theory** and **simulation theory**—both of which say that thinking about how other people think is an in-the-head matter. Shaun Gallagher advocates for **primary intersubjectivity** as the starting point for understanding others. This theory says that understanding others is a kind of embodied practice.

So while Gallagher can launch sharp criticisms at cognitivism, it's from far outside their own turf. It's hard to see how debate could get off the ground, since neither party grants the existence of the other's basic ontology.

10.5 Throwing out the baby with the bathwater?

A final worry for strong embodiment is that, at least as it is sometimes presented, we're throwing out an extensive set of concepts that are deeply rooted in the Western philosophical and scientific traditions. For example, in Sections 9.3.1 and 9.3.2, we suggested that you stop thinking about minds as things people have. But thinking about minds as things has a very long history in Western thought. We talk about beliefs and desires, for example, as states of mind. It's hard to see how you can have a state of mind if minds aren't things! If we go the route of strong embodiment, we lose many, if not all, of these concepts. If minds are not things, then we lose vast swathes of research in philosophy, psychology, neuroscience, linguistics, and more. Some philosophers suggest that this move is too drastic. Catherine Legg, for example, thinks that the concept of mental representation is useful, but it needs some serious overhauling to better fit with embodiment.

Some strong embodiment philosophers and scientists see the implication of strong embodiment and bite the bullet. Francisco Varela, Evan Thompson, and Eleanor Rosch, in their landmark book *The Embodied Mind*, have several chapters on Buddhism as a useful conversation partner for embodiment.[2] For many, that might be a bridge too far.

Notes

1 If you're interested in learning more about cognitive neuroscience, read Nichols and Newsome (1999) "The neurobiology of cognition."

2 Though in Thompson's and Rosch's introductions to the revised edition, published in 2016 (25 years after the initial publication), they offer some concerns about such conversations.

PART 3

Applications and extensions

11

INTERLUDE

Exposition to application

We've reached the end of our expository chapters. We've discussed disembodied views of mind, weak and strong views of embodiment, and criticisms of each. We've laughed. We've cried. Hopefully, we've all learned some important life lessons along the way.

11.1 Back to the metatheory

Remember from Chapter 5 how we outlined stress testing approaches:

	Stress testing approaches	
	What to do with iffy cases	*So things outside the head are...*
i. Optimist	It's either EM or it's not; we just have to do some more digging and figure it out.	Either constitutive *or* causal.
ii. Binary	Either everything is EM or nothing is	Either constitutive *or* causal.
iii. 2+ options	Create "subdivisions" based on certain conditions	Judged based on additional criteria (e.g., "Partly extended," if parity, but no coupling)
iv. Spectrum	Figure out where they lie on the spectrum between two extremes	Placed on a continuum between limit cases

DOI: 10.4324/9781003356622-14

How do weak and strong embodiment stack up here? Weak embodiment, as we've described it, gets the body into the mind by way of representations. Since the mechanisms of cognition are still in the head, weak embodiment takes the Binary approach and argues that *nothing* is EM. The mind doesn't extend out into the world.

But remember that weak embodiment is a functionalist view, which means it plays nicely with the Clark-style extended mind.[1] So the "extended" view of weak embodiment ends up falling into the Optimist category. There are genuine cases of extended mind, and further conceptual and empirical work can iron out iffy cases. So weak embodiment falls into the Binary approach; from there, whether things outside the head are causal or constitutional depends on your thoughts about the extended mind.

Now consider strong embodiment. Which approach does it take? Depending on how you spell out the details, you're looking at the Binary approach, 2+ options, or the Spectrum. Let's walk through the options.

First, you could take a really radical view of strong embodiment, which says that *everything* is EM, which is a version of the Binary approach. From this sort of view, cognition is always and everywhere extended. A useful slogan is: extended *because* embodied. It's because cognition is so deeply embodied and embedded in the world that all cases of cognition lean on the environment to some extent. It might be obvious, like when we use a smartphone to help us navigate. Or it might be more subtle, like when cultural influences shape how the world shows up for us. Some enactivists, like Alva Noë, Ezequiel di Paolo, Giovanna Colombetti, Pierre Steiner, and Hanne de Jaegher, are perhaps willing to endorse this. Similar comments go for some ecological psychologists, like JJ Gibson, and radically embodied cognitive scientists, like Tony Chemero, Ed Baggs, Sarah Bro Trasmundi, and Miguel Segundo-Ortin.

Next, consider the possibility of 2+ options. What might this look like? You have the categories of: causally related, constitutively related, and situated (as the in-between option). For example, you might agree that hearing a dog bark reminding me to take my dog for a walk is a case of a sound causing me to remember something. The bark is a cause, but it's not part of the cognitive system. You might also agree that my smartphone is part of my cognitive system. Finally, you might recognize that much of our activity is dependent on the environment, but the environment isn't part of the cognitive system. To remember to return my (CL) library books, I'll leave them by the front door. The presence of the books at the door reminds me that I need to return them. Neither the books nor the front door is part of the cognitive system, but both play a deeper role in my memory system than simply triggering a thought. My remembering is situated but not extended.

Or consider another case that arguably falls into the same extended-situated-causal buckets. Listening to certain songs reliably affects my emotions. Imagine you hear a song unexpectedly that triggers strong emotions, like joy, sadness, or nostalgia. While the song might reliably affect my emotional state, I didn't have any say in its coming on at that moment. It seems strange to say that the song is part of my cognitive system, but it seems less strange to say that the song is part of the cognitive context in which I'm currently situated.

In these cases, you end up with a strongly embodied view but one that's weaker than what we talked about in Chapter 9. There are some things that are definitely embodied without the need for representations, but there are other categories for which representations might be needed, like our book and song examples. We think that views in the second-wave extended mind (discussed in Chapter 6) from philosophers like Richard Menary and John Sutton fit in this category. Menary and Sutton both argue that some kinds of cognition don't require mental representations (e.g., skilled baseball players), but others do (e.g., imagining).

Consider, lastly, the Spectrum approach: there is a spectrum of positions between causal relations and constitutive relations in the cognitive system, and token instances of cognition fall somewhere on the scale. How do we determine where they fall? There might be some rough rules of thumb, but there aren't hard and fast rules. If there were, the Spectrum view would just be another version of the 2+ view.

One plausible way to interpret the Spectrum view is to say "we'll figure it out on a case-by-case basis." For example, suppose you use a calculator to figure out the value of 16/3 as part of your job (you need 1/3 cup of water and your cheap boss refuses to buy the measuring cup, claiming that you have tablespoons and teaspoons and that's good enough). You punch in the numbers and the function key and see that 16/3 = 5.33. You need 5 ⅓ tablespoons (i.e., five tablespoons and one teaspoon). You do this again and again until you just know that 16/3 is 5.33.

Suppose the next time you need to calculate 16/3, you whip out your calculator as a matter of habit, but you already know what it is. This last time of using the calculator *looks* just like every other time, but in this case, you didn't need it to give you the answer. One interpretation of this situation is that every instance of dividing 16 by 3 was a case of extended cognition *except* for the last one. In that final instance, where you knew the answer already, the cognition was happening "in the head." Here, the Spectrum view is helpful: all token instances of cognition are on the continuum. The first few were on the constitutive side of the spectrum, and the last few were on the causal side.

I'm not sure that there is any view that explicitly endorses this in the philosophical literature. What comes pretty close is a view from Andy Clark (2010). He argues that it doesn't really matter whether token cases of cognition are labelled as "extended" or not. What matters is wether the label helps move the sciences of mind forward. This would be his rule of thumb: if treating the case as extended proves scientifically fruitful, then it's a case of extended cognition.

11.2 The next section of the book

Now we're moving into what the different notions of embodiment mean for three areas: free will, ethics, and technology. There have been a lot of discussions about embodiment in consciousness studies, cognitive science, AI, and related fields. Basically, there's been a lot of work on embodiment in areas that are about mind. We (AK and CL) want to show that thinking carefully about embodiment matters for many areas of our lives. But why *these* three? The first two are issues that are covered in many introductory philosophy courses. Where I (CL) teach, students are required to take three philosophy classes, two of which cover issues in free will and ethics. Our goal to make this book accessible and useful; we want to connect ideas about embodiment to perennial philosophical issues. Additionally, thinking carefully about free will and ethics is, important.

Embodiment and technology are quickly becoming issues for all of us to think carefully about. Our situation is one of embodiment—that's just what we are. Technological developments are happening at incredible speeds. In our lifetimes, we (CL and AK) have gone from pagers as a novel technology to smart watches. Our parents grew up when computers were as big as rooms and slower than molasses. Now, people born in the 1950s can own a smartphone with more computational power (and for much cheaper) than computer scientists could have even dreamed of in the 1950s.

You're probably in your late-teens or early-to-mid-20s as you're reading this. The developments in technology you'll experience in the next 50 years will outstrip what we (CL and AK) imagined as possible. Thinking carefully about technology as it relates to our embodied situation is no luxury; it's a necessity as we lean on greater technological sophistication for our lives and livelihoods.

In the upcoming chapters, we'll consider each topic for both weak and strong embodiment. There's something we want to note now that will be clear as you continue reading. Weak and strong embodiment don't offer opposing answers to the same questions. They offer different ways of looking at the questions. For example, a common view leading up to questions around free will is that our beliefs and desires cause our actions: I want P and believe that not P unless Q; therefore, I want Q. (For example, I want ice cream but believe I won't have ice cream unless I go to the freezer. Therefore, I want to go to the freezer.) This way of conceptualizing the issue depends on a representational view of mind, which fits with weak embodiment. But if you don't have representations, how do we frame the problem? We won't tell you here, so you'll have to read on to find out.

Generally, here's how the chapters will proceed. First, we will lay out some of the big questions and positions in the field. Then, we ask, "given how the field has developed, what do theories of embodiment have to do with the standard questions and positions?" Lastly, we invert priority: we ask "given that we are embodied and embedded organisms, what kinds of questions do we have concerning free will (or ethics or technology)?"

Note

1 Recall that Clark-style extended mind is a functionalist view (see Section 7.7).

12

FREE WILL, DETERMINISM, AND EMBODIMENT*

12.1 Chapter overview

Here, we cover three views about the nature of free will and determinism: libertarianism (you are free and not determined), determinism (you are determined and not free), and compatibilism (you're both free and determined). We will first take those groupings of theories and suggest that embodiment offers some interesting complications to what seems fairly straightforward. For instance, if you think the mind extends beyond the body (see Chapter 4), then it's not easy to distinguish between individual and environment, which is typically presupposed in discussions about determinism and free will. But if we take our ideas about embodiment as fundamental, then new questions open up about the nature of agency and how to formulate questions about freedom in the first place.

12.2 Free will and determinism: the debate

You're reading this book. Is this a freely chosen action or is it determined? On the one hand, you might think that it's free. No one is holding a gun to your head (or at least we *really* hope not), and you're doing it because you have a desire to read it. Your professor might be the cause of the desire, but it's still *your* desire. That's all to say that you have chosen to read the book

* Many thanks to Avalyn Renee and Erik Inglis for conversations on the topics in this chapter during the course of their independent studies.

DOI: 10.4324/9781003356622-15

of your own volition. The act is free. Your **will**—that in virtue of which you are able to make choices—is free. Your act is free because you decide on your emotions, desires, and attitudes.

On the other hand, you're made up of bajillions of atomic and subatomic particles. These particles move according to the laws of physics. Think about one of Newton's laws of motion: an object in motion stays in motion unless something disrupts it. If an object is soaring through the air, some pretty basic math and physics will tell you where it will land and how long it will take. That's to say that physical objects are governed by physical laws. Since you're a physical object (i.e., you're made up of stuff that physicists study), you're governed by physical laws. Physical laws are deterministic: given a set of inputs, there is one output. So your choice is determined.

"But hold on," you reply. "I remember reading somewhere that some people think we are both free and determined." You're right; well done! It might be that you're determined to make a certain kind of choice given the sort of person you are. But also, you consider your options and make the choice you make. So in one way, you're determined; but in another way, you're free. Each of these is an option with associated arguments: libertarianism, determinism, and compatibilism. You can think of the overarching arguments like this:

> **Premise 1**: Either your behavior is determined or your actions are freely chosen.
> **Premise 2a**: Your behavior is *not* determined [libertarian premise]
> **Conclusion a**: Your actions are freely chosen [libertarian conclusion]
> **Premise 2b**: Your actions are *not* freely chosen [determinist premise]
> **Conclusion b**: Your actions are determined [determinist conclusion]

Conclusion *a* comes from Premise 1 and Premise 2a by the rule of disjunctive syllogism. Conclusion *b* comes from Premise 1 and Premise 2b by the same rule. The compatibilist responds by rejecting Premise 1: your behavior can be determined and your actions freely chosen. Let's get into it.

12.3 Libertarianism[1]: you are free

Think about what you've done so far today. Maybe you've eaten breakfast, gone to class (or work), fed the dog, washed the dishes, or taken a shower. Some of these you can do on autopilot, but you have to make a choice to do them. It doesn't take a lot of attention to shower, but you can choose to shower or not. Being able to choose to do X or not is characteristic of a lot of our activities. I (CL) am typing this chapter. I could be doing something else, like going to the bar or watching TV.

There are a lot of things that we do that are involuntary. For example, after you eat a sandwich, your stomach digests the food. When you stub your toe, you wince in pain. We blink, breathe, and barf largely without our choosing to do so. There's a lot that goes on without our choosing it. We're excluding those sorts of behaviors from our consideration.

So why think that we're free? In a way, it kind of seems obvious. If you walk out of the room and your friend asks why you're leaving, you can give them a response, like, "I'm hungry." More generally, we can answer "why" questions by describing our reasons for doing something. If we refrained from performing an action—like I didn't jump off a cliff while all of my friends did[2]—we can offer reasons for why we didn't do the thing. In these cases and many others like them, it's you or me or whoever that performs the action because of a willingness to do so. It just *seems* like we're free.[3]

Of course, it seems like there are some things we do that are *not* free. If you're mugged at gunpoint, you don't have a choice to hand over your wallet.[4] Or if you get on the bus and the bus driver goes rogue and takes me away from my place of work, then you did not freely choose to be late to work. In these cases, you are coerced. It might be hard to find the boundary between "freely chosen" and "coerced." Suppose instead of a gun, someone threatens to beat you up to get your wallet. Suppose further that you are the famed boxer Mike Tyson. Odds are, you could successfully fight this person and keep your wallet, but you hand over your wallet. Were you coerced?

Another reason to think why we're free: our entire legal system and society depend on it. There are (at least) two situations in which someone isn't held responsible for their actions: if they were forced or if they didn't know what they were doing (their doing X resulted in Y, which they couldn't have foreseen/known about). In the case of being forced, it's clear that the person who is coerced into the action didn't choose to do it freely. As a result, they are not held liable. Now in the case of a person who performed an action but was not aware that they did whatever it is that they did, their lack of knowledge about the circumstances or the outcomes prevents them from having chosen to perform that action or bring about that outcome. Since they did not choose to perform that action, they're not held liable for it. So, the argument goes, we have a kind of practical necessity to believe that we are free. Additionally, the argument goes, we can't even make sense of the idea of responsibility unless we are free. So in addition to the practical necessity of believing that we are free, our very idea for responsibility depends on our being free.

Now, the libertarian has an important task they have to complete. They have to offer some kind of ontology or metaphysics as part of the idea that we are free. The reason why this is such a challenge is because it would seem, given the arguments above about the physical world, that we are not free. The strategy for the libertarian is to describe the relationship between minds and the world in such a way that choices we make are not constrained by physical facts of the world.

One way is found in Descartes. Descartes posited that we are disembodied, and that means that you and me and any other person you know don't exist in the physical world. Remember, to be disembodied for Descartes is to have an immaterial mind that exists outside the physical world. And since you, the thing that chooses and decides on a course of action, exist outside the physical world, then you are not constrained by the laws of physics. And for all of the criticisms we levied against the disembodied view of mind, this is one distinct advantage. If the mind is disembodied and not determined by the laws of nature, then we have an easy and intuitive explanation for how we are free.

Nonetheless, if you are not a fan of disembodied minds or of Descartes, there is another strategy. This is one found in the work of Roderick Chisholm. Chisholm distinguished between two kinds of causal relationships. The first is **transeunt causation**. This is a kind of causal relationship between **events**. Events can be philosophically tricky to specify, but a handy way to think about them is as goings-on that begin with a verb ending in "ing." Here are some examples: closing the door, opening the refrigerator, voting for president, jumping up and down, cooking dinner, and raising your hand in class to ask a question. In general, you can think about this as one state of affairs causing another state of affairs. This is intuitively different from a different kind of causal relationship, **immanent causation**. Immanent causation is when an agent brings about some state affairs. So we mentioned raising your hand in class in the previous sentence, but what brings about the raising of your hand in class to ask a question? It is you, the person, who brings about those states of affairs. Immanent causation, because it is initiated by the person, is not determined. We *can*, of course, provide a description of one state of affairs in your brain causing the raising of your hand; but this description misses an important generalization about causes. Namely, that agent-level causes are used to assess responsibility.

The more you know: Typically, when we think about cause and effect, we think of examples like a baseball bat hitting a ball and the ball flying off into left field, or turning on the light switch and the light coming on. This is known as **efficient causation**. The term comes from Aristotle, and was one of the four different kinds of causes that he argued in favor of. Another kind of causal relationship that Aristotle identified is known as **final causation**. This is a kind of causal relationship where we think about something's goal or purpose. This is easiest to see with people. When we inquire into the reason or the purpose of somebody's doing something, we are asking about their goal. The goal state is the final cause for the behavior. Jumping ahead a few millennia, it's common to distinguish between **proximal causes** and **distal causes**. Proximal causes are causes that are close to the outcome in space and time. So when I eat a dish consisting of garlic and onions, my hunger is the proximal cause for my action. Distal causes are causes that are further away in space and time. A distal cause of my eating that dish might be some kind of evolutionary disposition. In fact, some psychologists and anthropologists find that garlic and onions are a common combination in many parts of the world, so there might be some kind of beneficial biological effect provided by that combination.

These are just a few different ideas about causal relationships that you can find in philosophy. The reason why we want to introduce them is because we find that students have a tendency to think of all causes as efficient causation. But if you think that all causes are efficient causes, you miss out on important generalizations about the world. An intuitive example is the presence of wealth disparities among races in the United States. Many cities practiced redlining, which prohibited non-white citizens from buying homes in parts of cities. When home values were assessed, it may be no surprise that the homes in non-white neighborhoods were valued lower than homes in predominantly white neighborhoods. This has had a cumulative effect over generations, enabling *on average* white families to have greater wealth than non-white families. So when thinking about the causes for wealth disparities in the 21st century, thinking about redlining as an efficient cause doesn't fit very well.[5]

We have seen two different ways of preserving free will in the face of the indifferent determinism of the laws of nature. One is to remove the agent—the mind—from the physical world. The other is to provide a description of the events that satisfies an important explanatory interest.

12.4 Determinism: you are not free

We have seen some reasons to think that you are free. And now, we're going to consider some reasons to think that you are not free. In other words, we are going to consider how you might be determined and what that could mean.

We've seen one reason already for thinking that there is no such thing as free will. We are physical entities, and physical entities are governed by the laws of nature. So it follows that we also are governed by the laws of nature. And if we are governed by the laws of nature, then everything we do is determined by those laws and the initial state of the universe. This thought experiment goes back to a philosopher and scientist named **Pierre LaPlace**. The thought experiment is this. Imagine you knew all of the physical facts about the initial state of the universe and also imagine that you have complete knowledge of the laws of nature. With these two things, you could predict all future states of the universe. You would apply the relevant laws to the initial state. You would apply those same laws to any following states. So what you're doing now and where you are is the product of indifferent laws of nature guiding states of the universe.

The intuition behind this thought experiment is that if we know how the universe is at any point and we know the rules behind how the universe changes from one moment to the next, then we can predict future states of the universe.

The more you know: You might have noticed that the thought experiment was put in terms of knowledge. You have to know the initial state of the universe and you have to know the laws of nature. It's important to note that knowing something and that something being the way it is are two separate questions. Now one reason why we do this is to make the thought experiment feel more natural, but the hard work is being done by our conception of laws of nature. We can think about them as conditionals. If event A happens then event B happens. As an example, if water is heated to 100° C, then it will boil. What this is saying is that boiling is determined by the heating of the water.

This is one kind of determinism, and we think it's the one that comes to mind most readily when folks are thinking about how the universe and human behavior are determined. But there is another variety of determinism, called **psychological determinism**. We find this in the work of David

Hume. Psychological determinism claims that mental states and behaviors are determined by previous mental states. There are a couple of ways that we might imagine this. One way is in terms of our actions. Hume argues that our actions flow from our character. In other words, the kind of person we are and what our personalities are like determine the kinds of actions we perform. So our behaviors are determined by our personalities. Additionally, what we think and want is determined by our previous perceptions and mental states. So if I want an ice cream sandwich and believe that I won't have an ice cream sandwich unless I go to the grocery store, then I will go to the grocery store.

We saw previously that one of the benefits of the libertarian position is that it (i) fits with our experience of ourselves as free and (ii) makes sense of our practices of holding people responsible. So how can the determinist cope with these concerns?

With respect to the first point, the determinist would simply point out that our experience is often misleading. It seems to us as if the sun is moving across the sky, but in reality it's we who are moving and the sun that is staying still. So we might experience ourselves as free, but this is just another misleading perception.

With respect to the second point, one strategy is to use an analogical argument. Derk Pereboom offers the following in his essay "Free Will Skepticism and Criminal Punishment." Imagine someone who is ill and needs to be quarantined. Now this person didn't do anything to deserve being quarantined. Even so, for the sake of the community, the person is put into isolation so that others aren't infected. The lesson then is that people can be isolated even though they didn't do anything to deserve it. This lesson carries over into the case of crime. The person who is incarcerated may have been determined to commit their crime. But just as we quarantine the sick person, we "quarantine" people who have committed crimes. It's just that in the case of quarantining people who commit crimes, we falsely tell a narrative of how that person could have done otherwise. But in both cases, we isolate one person from the community for the benefit of the community.

The upshot to this approach is that it lets us have our determinism and also justify punishment. The trade-off is that people aren't punished because of something they chose to do. Responsibility is no longer a matter of people's individual choices.

12.5 Incompatibilism and compatibilism

Now, both the libertarian and determinist positions assume that free will and determinism are incompatible. That is, if one is true, then the other must be false. This is known as **incompatibilism**. Incompatibilism seems intuitively true, but what are some reasons to believe it?

The philosopher Peter van Inwagen offers one argument. It is detailed, but we will just look at the highlights here. He begins by observing that there is nothing we can do to change the past. Also, there is nothing we can do to change the laws of nature. From these two points, he infers that all of our actions are the necessary consequences of what happened in the past and the laws of nature. In other words, there is nothing we can do about our present actions. We are unable to do anything other than what we have done and what we are doing. But free will seems to require that we could have done something differently. Therefore, if determinism is true, we could not have acted differently and we do not have free will. And if we have free will, then we could have done things differently and determinism is false. Van Inwagen concludes that you can have one or the other but not both.

Contrary to this, there is a robust tradition in the history of Western philosophy that free will and determinism are compatible. This is called **compatibilism**. One version of compatibilism, which has come to be known as **classical compatibilism**, makes two claims about what it means to act freely. One is that we have the power or ability to do whatever it is we want to do. This doesn't mean that you always act on those desires, but it just means that you have the ability to act on certain desires. Second, you are not constrained or coerced into acting or not. We saw an example of coercion above: being forced into doing something at gunpoint. In that case, you do not act freely because you are coerced. But you can likewise be constrained in a number of ways. For example, if you are temporarily paralyzed or if the resources available to you to complete some task are insufficient, these are again examples in which you do not act freely or you cannot act freely.

At the same time, you are determined; not only that, but we *need* determinism in order to make sense of free will. Suppose you give your sandwich to your friend because they forgot their lunch. You had a motive for doing this: you are generous and want to help your friend. Your motive is the cause of your action; your motive caused the generous behavior. If we didn't have these kinds of causal relationships between motives and actions, then we could never make sense of others' actions because we wouldn't have a reliable connection between cause (motive) and effect (behavior). So no one coerced you into giving your friend your sandwich; that is, you chose to give it to your friend. And also, you gave your friend your sandwich because you had a motivation to do so (i.e., generosity and compassion for your friend). Your motive caused you to give your friend the sandwich, and you chose to give your friend the sandwich.[6]

12.6 Free will and embodiment

That's the crash course introduction to the debate of free will and determinism. The big question is: how is embodiment related to all of this? We're going to tackle this in two parts. First, given the problem of free will and determinism, how does embodiment contribute to the debate? Second, given our embodiment, how does that shape the kinds of questions we ask about free will and determinism?

12.6.1 Freedom of action and freedom of will

We'll need a few more concepts to consider how ideas about embodiment contribute to questions about free will and determinism. Our first step is to distinguish between two kinds of freedom: **freedom of action** and **freedom of will**. Freedom of action is about being able to choose an action from among a range of possibilities. For example, freedom of action is being free to choose between taking the bus to work or driving or between oatmeal or toast for breakfast. These are the kinds of small, daily decisions we make. They're boring, but it's the stuff of everyday life. You can choose among actions that express your will (i.e., your emotions, attitudes, and desires).

Being able to choose your actions doesn't entail that you can choose your will. It could be that you have no control over your will, but you do have control over your actions. Freedom of will is a kind of freedom to form your own desires, emotions, and attitudes. It's a freedom to choose your desires. Harry Frankfurt, for example, says that while many animals have desires and make choices, only humans can form their desires based on other kinds of desires. You not only *want* something, but you *want to want* something. It's easy to see this with addiction behaviors. An alcoholic wants to consume alcohol, but they might wish that they didn't have this desire. They *want* alcohol, but they might have a desire to abstain from alcohol.[7]

To see the difference, consider the work of the behaviorist B.F. Skinner. He sometimes wrote about designing cultures to resemble utopian worlds. He has a novel about it, *Walden Two*, and he has a chapter devoted to it in his book *Science and Human Behavior*. The gist is that cultures are "experiments in behavior" and that we could live far better lives if we treated these cultures like controlled experiments: figure out what kinds of behaviors make for the best sorts of lives and then institute those changes. In *Walden Two*, for example, people in the community are divided into occupational groups. Some folks are planners, others are scientists, others are workers, and still others are managers. Some of the jobs for workers are physically strenuous, like being a laborer or doing trash pickup. To compensate for the greater difficulty of their labor, workers in especially taxing jobs would earn more "credits," like having more vacation days, than people with less taxing jobs. While being a garbage collector is hard, there are benefits. Now, the important thing for our purposes is that people make choices in the community on their own; there is no top-down imposition of a government's will. But the choices they make are conditioned by cultural engineering. In this sense, people can make choices, but their choices are constrained by the imposed social structure. There are choices *within* the society, but there's no choosing their will because society has been engineered in a way to form their wills for them. They have freedom of action—they can choose their breakfast—but not freedom of will.

12.6.2 Agency

Agency is one of those concepts that philosophers argue about a lot, but here's the rough idea. Agency is the feature of **persons** that enables them to be the authors of their lives within the constraints of their material reality. To say that you have agency is to say that you have control of your life, or at least control of some aspects of your life.

> **Otto's workbook**: You might have noticed the use of "person" in the previous paragraph. Personhood is a philosophical concept. It asks the question: what is it that makes something a *person*? This is a lot trickier than it seems. CL and AK are both persons. You reading this are likely a person. But, if this book is "read" by an artificial intelligence (e.g. a large language model), is that thing a person? The issue is an important one because it's believed that persons are things that *definitely* have moral rights. Persons have moral standing. Water bottles and rocks definitely do not have moral rights. In 250 words, describe some cases where it's questionable whether something is a person or not and explain why the case you've identified is a gray-area case.

"Agency" often carries with it social, economic, and political concerns. In other words, when we're thinking about the notion of agency, we're thinking about the capacities of an individual situated in a wider social world.

The more you know: There is a pair of concepts in philosophy that are helpful in distinguishing the difference between free will and agency: **narrow individuation** and **wide individuation**. "Individuate" means how we distinguish one thing from another. You can relate it to the word "individual": what are our criteria for marking one individual as different from another? Suppose you had two copies of *The Little Engine That Could*. In one sense, you have two different books since each one stands in different physical relationships to other things: One copy is closer to your stove than another. In another sense, it's the same book: what's between the pages is the same. (Just think, if you saw a copy of *The Little Engine That Could* on your friend's bookshelf, you could reasonably say, "Hey, I have the same book!") When we mark one thing as different from another solely in terms of features of those things (e.g. the contents of the book), we individuate *narrowly*. When we mark one thing as different from another in terms of relational features (e.g. how far one of the books is from some other object), we individuate *widely*.

This might be a helpful way to think about the difference between free will and agency. Often, when we're thinking about free will, we're thinking about our capacities *narrowly* in terms of our biology and mental states. Often, when we're thinking about agency, we're thinking about our capacities *widely* in terms of social structures and cultural institutions. It's important to note that this is a general rule but has its exceptions. For instance Galen Strawson, in his essay "The Impossibility of Ultimate Moral Responsibility" includes culture as part of his argument for the impossibility of ultimate moral responsibility, i.e. a sort of "the buck stops here" kind of responsibility.

12.7 Freedom of action, freedom of will, and embodiment

Consider again the framework in which we placed our discussion of freedom of action. The debate was about whether or not the choices we make are causally determined. The determinist says that our choices are determined by forces outside of our control, and therefore, we are not free. The libertarian says that people remain somewhere in the causal chain, and so our actions are free. The debate then comes down to the involvement of embodiment as we're thinking about the causal mechanisms involved in behavior.

12.7.1 Mental representations and freedom of action

Let's begin by considering some of the conceptual resources of weak embodiment. Recall that weak embodiment theorists believe that our mental representations are modal in character. That is, our thoughts might be about whatever, but they are often structured by the body.

When we think about weak embodiment in this way, it seems like the questions about free will and determinism that we've been considering so far carry over into discussions involving embodiment. So if the ontology for debates about free will and determinism is given in terms of mental representations or neurons, then weak embodiment slips into those debates without disturbing anything.

To see this, consider again the reasons that the determinist offers for their position. We are physical things in a physical universe, and consequently, we are governed by physical laws. Mental representations, insofar as they are realized in some material substance, are likewise governed by those physical laws. It doesn't really matter whether those are modal or amodal representations. Either way, they are realized in neural tissue or some physical substance.

However, adopting weak embodiment does put some constraints on our ideas of free will and determinism. If we are weakly embodied, then only humans can think or be free as humans are; animals and machines can't be free in the way that we are free. Consider that our modal representations are structured by sensory modalities, and sensory modalities are species specific. Our non-human, primate brethren also have binocular vision and stand upright at least sometimes. But our sensory apparatus is nonetheless a bit different from theirs. At the very least, we can perceive how some objects are socially meaningful and chimpanzees cannot. Children learn to read texts, but so far, the evidence suggests that chimpanzees cannot. It seems reasonable to suppose that this difference shows up in small ways in our visual systems, including not just the eyes but also the optic nerve and visual cortex. It also follows that if we are ever to build sophisticated enough machines, they could not be free in the same way that we are. Such sophisticated machines would be able to do a lot, we can imagine, but since they don't have human bodies, they wouldn't have the kinds of mental representations that we have. You might recall an objection from Ned Block along these lines. He noted that one of the problems with functionalism is that taking a chauvinist view means withholding attributions of mental states to systems that reasonably have them. But it's not clear that non-human systems are free in the same ways that we are. So in order for the objection to succeed, we'd have to have a good reason to think that machines and animals have free will.

Some have recently argued that free will is a reason to think that there *have* to be mental representations, which fits very well with weak embodiment. That is, the fact that we are free—that we are agents—means that there must be mental representations. The argument goes back to our introduction of representation-hungry activities from Section 10.4. Think for a moment about planning for the future, like planning your dinner for the evening. Thoughts about the future are thoughts about currently non-existent states of the world. After all, the dinner you're planning to make doesn't exist yet. But thinking about abstract entities requires mental representations. It's a representation-hungry activity. So since we can plan a future course of action, we must have mental representations, and weak embodiment is the better theory.

12.7.2 Extended minds and freedom of action

But there's yet another dimension to thinking about freedom of action. Remember the main theme of our jazz standard: extended cognition. Resources outside of the body to which we are reliably coupled are part of our cognitive system. So, how does this affect our freedom of action?

Once we begin to see that external props are part of the cognitive system, what "we" can do expands greatly. So, for example, the calculator on my phone does a lot of math for me. I can calculate a tip or figure out how much everyone has to chip in for the pizza because I have my phone. I couldn't figure that out on my own without my phone. And the more external resources to which I'm reliably coupled, the more I can do.

Now, what about the external resources to which I am *not* coupled? Do those things expand the range of activities I can accomplish? Do situational resources increase my freedoms of action? For example, I have reliable access to an oven in my kitchen. Does having that increase, decrease, or not affect my freedoms of action? Consider it for a moment before we tell you what we think.

> **Otto's workbook**: Consider some other examples of situational resources expanding what you're capable of doing, like a car, bicycle, ladder, or scissors. Does having or losing these things affect your freedoms of action? Why or why not?

This is an interesting question (we think, at least) because freedom of action is often thought of in narrow terms. You are free insofar as you have the mental and physical capability to do one thing or another. The external world enters the story insofar as the situational resources are props or things for you to use as you're going about your day, doing stuff. When we ask if you're more free when you have external resources with which to accomplish a variety of tasks, typically the emphasis is on the on-board resources—your body and mind. Asking if you're more free when you have a bicycle is a bit like saying "if I had a bicycle, I could do such-and-such." You're free to do what you like within your means and if you had more means you could do more things. This way of thinking about freedom of action and cognitive situatedness treats the availability of cognitive resources as a merely contingent variable. Of course, you could bake a cake if you had an oven! But the availability of the oven to you doesn't affect how we think about your freedoms of action. Your freedoms are about *you*, not what's available to you.

However, what if we *do* think about your freedoms of action as contingent on what resources are available to you in your environment? In other words, what if we think about how free you are as changing over time and circumstance? For starters, what you're free to do would be context-dependent—you're more free *sometimes* and *somewheres* than others. Your freedoms of action are more constrained in some environments than others. Some people have more freedoms than others. For example, one way of thinking about fines for breaking the law is that the fines are just part of the cost of doing whatever you like. After all, you can park wherever you like as long as you don't mind paying a fine.

Now, if we think about our freedoms of action as being importantly tied to situational resources, then you are more or less free, given the circumstances of your life. When you say you can't (let's suppose) go to Paris for the weekend because you don't have the money, that is a literal constraint on your freedoms. Someone who can drop that kind of cash is literally freer than you are.

This is interesting because questions of free will are usually thought of as purely metaphysical and not touching the social, political, or economic domains. In fact, that's exactly what we find in Descartes's *Meditations on First Philosophy*. He describes people as being as free as they could possibly be. In fact, our will—our capacity to choose—is our most God-like capacity, according to Descartes. We are all equally free in Descartes's view, but our circumstances differ. But if minds are extended or situated, then we are not equally free.

There are also interesting moral applications too. Consider a line from "Mathematics" from the rapper Mos Def: "When the average minimum wage is $5.15//You best believe you gotta find new ground to get C.R.E.A.M."[8] Mos Def here bemoans the state of young African-American men, sometimes turning to dangerous means to earn money, notably selling drugs and expanding one's selling area (i.e., "new ground") to do so. If our freedom of action is partly constituted by the situating environment, there could be a literal sense in which some people are unable to do otherwise.

Side quest: The philosopher **Harry Frankfurt** is known for devising a category of cases that challenge the **Principle of Alternate Possibilities:** someone is morally responsible for an action only if they could have done otherwise. (This principle is often taken as an argument against the compatibility of determinism and moral responsibility.) In a 1000-word essay, (i) explain such a Frankfurt case and (ii) how it bears on the discussion of extended/situated cognition and freedom of action.

12.7.3 Freedom of will and constraining desires

Much of what we've said carries over into thinking about freedom of will: being able to choose the state of your will. What's the connection? Think about your will as the cause of the actions you perform. Questions about embodiment and the will are about the relationship between being embodied and your capacity to choose your desires. So the basic framework stays the same, but there are nonetheless many interesting issues.

One is the idea of a Ulysses contract. In *The Odyssey*, the main character Ulysses (aka Odysseus) wants to hear the song of the Sirens. The upside to hearing the song is that their voices are beautiful. The downside is that it will kill you. Their song makes hearers lose all rational thought, jumping into the sea (and drowning) in an attempt to join them. Ulysses has his men tie him to the mast and then fill their ears with wax so they cannot hear their song. He instructs them to keep him tied up no matter how much he begs to be released. Ulysses creates a condition that constrains his future choices.

We do this all the time: you might avoid buying cookies so you're not able to eat the cookies. But we can also do this with our wills: we can create conditions that shape our wills. Suppose you find yourself consuming more alcohol (or smoking or watching TV or whatever) than you like. Now you *want* to consume alcohol, but you want to want to consume less alcohol. What can you do? You can create the conditions to shape your will. You might avoid going to the bar or spend less time with friends who consume a lot of alcohol. In doing this, you not only consume less alcohol but you also reduce your desire to consume alcohol. That is, by doing these things, you shape your will.

12.8 Rethinking agency and free will

One powerful aspect of a strongly embodied approach to thinking about free will is that it can encourage us to reframe how we think about free will and human agency—that is given that we are embodied, new questions about agency and free will open up. To have agency is to be able to become the sort of person you want to be and to do the sorts of things you want to do. A related concept is **autonomy**. To be autonomous is to be self-determining. The term comes from two Greek words: *auto*, meaning "self" and *nomos*, meaning "law." To be autonomous is to be self-legislating, a giver of laws to oneself. Questions of agency and autonomy typically bracket issues about being determined by natural laws.[9] Issues of agency and autonomy often take on social and political dimensions. For example, suppose you're a woman in the 1950s and you wish to get a divorce. You could, but you'd have to show wrongdoing by your husband, which can be difficult depending on the nature of the relationship.[10] This law limited the agency of women in the United States: they were unable, because of social structures, to exercise their agency to leave their husbands.

When we think about free will, we often adopt a narrow perspective. We think about our bodies and our minds. From this narrow perspective, freedom is a kind of rugged individualism. It's *you* who are free, and freedom means not relying on others. This is **individualistic autonomy**. Our ability to act freely and choose our own paths has nothing to do with others. Your agency begins and ends with you.

Side quest: This notion of autonomy is culture-bound. Western cultures—like the US, the UK, and Canada—are highly individualistic and often default to thinking of autonomy as individualistic because the self is individualistic. The cultural psychologist Geert Hofstede has an excellent set of resources on his website: https://geerthofstede.com. In particular, navigate to the page discussing the 6-D model of national culture and watch a short video of Hofstede discussing individualism and collectivism. What are the differences between individualistic and collectivist views of the self and their implications for conceptions of autonomy?

But that's not the only way to think about autonomy. We can also think about agency as the kinds of choices we can make with respect to possibilities available to us in a given economic, social, cultural, and political landscape. Free will and agency, on this view, aren't *only* matters of what's in our heads or how the mind is connected to the body. It's about how we're connected to the wider world and each other. This kind of autonomy is called **relational autonomy**. A great place to begin reading about relational autonomy is Catriona Mackenzie's essay "Relational Autonomy."

Before we give you a flavor of this research, a heads up that, even within this niche of a niche of a niche, we can't cover everything. Issues about agency and the body have been explored extensively in feminist philosophy and phenomenology. Much of what we discuss in this section comes from the work of philosophers like Diana Tietjens Meyers, Iris Marion Young, Nancy Tuana, and Lorraine Code. We'll offer some guides to the very rich literature, but the best way to learn more about it is to dive in.

Our point of departure is to recognize that talk of freedom and autonomy occurs at different timescales. (We introduced talk about timescales in the chapter on strong embodied cognition.) When asking the question of whether we're free or determined in terms of brain activity, we're at the level of milliseconds. And even taking evolutionary and personal history into account, we're still thinking about what's happening in the brain: how have evolutionary and ontogenetic histories shaped how our brains work?

Those are fair questions, but we can also ask about freedom and autonomy at a different timescale: days, weeks, months, years, decades, centuries. Insofar as autonomy is in some way social, then we use timescales appropriate to social organisms like ourselves. Consider, for a moment, the pressure exerted on women to satisfy beauty norms, otherwise known as the **male gaze.** In 2022, women in the USA underwent 25.1 million cosmetic procedures, ranging from breast enhancement and reduction to liposuction to eyelid surgery. (Men underwent roughly 1.4 million procedures.) Patients in that year spent over $26 billion on these surgeries. When we think about the time and money spent on satisfying cultural norms of beauty, it seems natural to ask "why?" Some of these procedures are minor and noninvasive, but others are spendy and have a moderately painful recovery. The obvious answer is that these women (and some men) want to look better; they want to be more attractive.[11] But there's a question hot on the heels of this answer: why do women want to be perceived as more conventionally attractive? One plausible answer is because of cultural norms about beauty. Culture tells a story about how women *ought* to look, and many do their best to live up to that narrative. In a sense, then, women's autonomy in certain respects is impinged upon as a result of internalized cultural norms. On this line of thought, women aren't free to appear however they like; how women appear and want to appear is governed by cultural norms.

Side quest: One response to the above line of reasoning is, "but there are many women who conscientiously reject social norms of appearance. How are we to think about such cases?" (A hint to point you towards one possible response is an old saying about the massively influential philosopher **Immanuel Kant:** You can philosophize with Kant, or philosophize against him, but you cannot philosophize without him. How might a similar sentiment apply?)

We've argued our point about agency and social rules using beauty standards for women, but the general point applies to any social or cultural norms that are prevalent enough in the population to inform choices and judgments.

Otto's workbook: Come up with two of your own examples of internalized norms that constrain the actions and judgments of a group.

On a strongly embodied approach, the major conceptual shift is in the constraints on our actions. We are to look at how embodied entities living in social and cultural contexts are constrained by those contexts. When we adopt this perspective, we get a new and interesting range of questions. For example, consider the Greensboro lunch counter sit-ins during the American Civil Rights movement, which happened in 1960 in North Carolina.[12] It started with four African-American men sitting at a lunch counter in protest. There were no *laws* prohibiting it, but there were very strong social norms (sometimes backed with the threat of violence) enforcing segregation.[13] Arguably, African-Americans weren't free to sit at the lunch counters in previous years, say in 1950. But if they weren't free to sit at lunch counters in 1950, how could those four African-American students have done it 10 years later? How did members of a race become "more free"? Explanations will have to include historical, socio-cultural, and personal forces. For instance, the Greensboro sit-in wasn't the first of its kind, though it is among the more famous. For example, there was a sit-in at a library in Virginia[14] in 1939, and this historical precedent might have made the action seem more possible. Also, segregation was outlawed in 1954 in *Brown v. Board of Education*. There were also *four* students—a *single* student may not have been free to do it. And finally, the four students may have had strong beliefs that others would join them in their cause, which turned out to be exactly right. The upshot is that freedom and free will aren't discovered by turning to our species' biological history or God or the Big Bang. Instead, we are to look at the social and cultural institutions that support or constrain our freedom. Questions of agency are about embodied and embedded agents and what they can or cannot do.

Side quest: Someone (likely a philosopher) might point out that the students were free the entire time. What changed was their *beliefs* about what they could do. So we don't need to look to social and cultural institutions and structures to learn more about autonomy. We would be much better off looking at what people believe about those institutions and structures. What do you think of this objection? Do you agree or disagree? Either way, what reasons do you have for your position?

We might refer to this as **freedom of opportunity**. While freedom of action and freedom of will focus narrowly on the individual, freedom of opportunity focuses on the situated agent. If we consider a social prohibition on some action—but it can be physically performed by the agent in question—we are looking at a constraint on freedoms of opportunity. For example, I often note to my students that they could easily gang up on me and overtake me by force if they didn't like their grades on a test. (Fortunately, no one has put this to the test.) So while my students have the freedom of action to overpower me, they do not have the freedom of opportunity to do so.

12.9 Agency, embodiment, and expertise

Consider for a moment something you do habitually—drive a car, ride a bicycle, wash dishes, type, drink a cup of coffee, tie your shoes, or put on pants. In each of these cases and many more, you don't think about what you're doing. When you were first learning to tie your shoes, you focused on holding the laces just right and wrapping the loops around one another in the right ways. This kind of action and thought is slow and deliberative. Now, you just tie your shoes. You don't have to pay attention in the same way as when you were learning to tie them. It might sound odd, but you're an expert at shoe-tying. These are activities that required focus and attention at one point, but now can be done on autopilot. They have become habitual.

Let's up the ante. Think of activities like reading, playing chess, or interpreting some empirical data. These are very clearly cognitive activities, but they are habits just like shoe-tying. Consider, for example, how to interpret empirical data. Doing this requires a degree of skill. Some schmo off the street can't reliably interpret data. It takes someone with training and expertise. Such a person exercises their expertise in interpreting the data. Importantly, they don't reflect on the activity of interpreting the data as they interpret the data. Just as the expert car driver drives their car without reflecting on how they drive their car, expert scientists interpret the data without reflecting on how they interpret their data.

Now, they *might* reflect on their practices at some point in the future. Suppose you keep getting into accidents as you're driving. You might start to pay attention to your driving habits so that you get into fewer accidents. In these moments when you're reflecting on your expert performance, you aren't acting in the role of expert. You're thinking about how to perform in your role as an expert.

Hubert Dreyfus, a philosopher who has thought through issues of expertise extensively, argues that when any of us is engaged in activities that we can do on "autopilot," we are not thinking or reflecting on what we're doing. We're simply acting. We're doing the things we know how to do. That's easy to see in cases like driving or going down a rabbit hole on Wikipedia. You don't have to think about how you're doing it; you're just doing it. But when we're learning a skill, we have to think about how we're performing the action. When you learn to ride a bike, you have to pay close attention to how your body is moving and how to maintain your balance. There's a lot to keep track of! But as you get more skilled at riding a bike, the less you think about how to ride. Similarly, folks who have lost a leg will sometimes have it replaced by a running blade. The more they run with the running blades, the more skilled they become at it until they don't think about it at all.

Dreyfus claims that the same thing goes for cognitive activities too. Consider playing chess—surely a cognitive activity if anything is. When you're learning to play chess, you're thinking hard and trying to remember which pieces move in what ways. With practice, you can move the pieces without thinking about the rules. At this point, you start to think about strategy. Early learners will often have a strategy of capturing as many pieces as they can. This can work sometimes, but getting more skilled in chess requires better strategies. At this point, the novice reflects on how they think about moves to make. They practice predicting what the other player will do. The more they do this, the better they get at it. Eventually, thinking about what the other player is thinking about becomes second nature. From here, you might advance to thinking about how particular players make their choices. So you're not just predicting the other person's moves; you're predicting how Smith or Jones will move.

The point, Dreyfus argues, is that everyday expertise is a better model for thinking about human cognition. Expertise in these multitudes of ways represents the majority of what we do. Each of these complex tasks had to be learned and perfected. Of course, we can reflect on our performance, but typically, we're engaged in the performance. This may sound very similar from Chapter 9 on strong embodied cognition. Everyday, embodied expertise is far more representative of our problem solving than word puzzles or math problems.

So how does this tie back into agency? When we develop expertise, we both expand and constrain our agency. We expand agency by developing a set of skills that enable us to do certain kinds of things we weren't able to do before. When you're an expert chess player, you can now do things you couldn't do before, like take on other expert chess players. But your agency is also constrained: certain moves aren't available to you anymore. Analogously, it can be difficult for professional singers to intentionally sing off-key because they have honed their capacities to sing on-key.

Another important point is that we have to think carefully about how and why we attribute moral responsibility. In the USA, there's a burden of proof (in some cases) to show that the defendant *intended* to commit the crime. Sometimes, this might be easy: if there's a paper trail of planning that specifies how the crime was to be committed, for instance. Other times, it might be hard. Suppose you find yourself in an altercation—heated words are being exchanged, tempers are beginning to flare. If you push the other person and they are seriously injured as a result, you—literally—might not have been thinking about the action as you performed it. You were acting with a kind of expertise. You might notice in hindsight that your action was dangerous; that is, you might reflect and understand for yourself that the action was dangerous. This isn't to say that you shouldn't be held morally responsible—maybe you should. But what we're trying to point out is this: that in virtue of which we assign blame may be a *lot* more complicated than whether someone meant to do something.

12.10 Wrapping up the chapter

12.10.1 Embodiment's contribution to positions considering free will and determinism

As (we hope) is clear, the notion of embodiment can, but doesn't have to, play an important role in thinking about free will. Of course, the ways in which perennial topics are discussed ebb and flow. Embodiment has sometimes been important in thinking about free will and autonomy, and sometimes hasn't.

The way in which embodiment can matter depends on which flavor of embodiment strikes you as more plausible. Weak embodiment focuses on freedoms of action and helps to make questions about determinism more precise. It's not that the brain sends impulses to various parts of the body, which then carry out the command. Instead, the "higher" cognitive functions of the brain are informed by and inform the "lower" functions. Thinking about kicking a ball lights up parts of the brain that have to do with flinging your leg. So instead of thinking of the causal sequence as,

1 Brain activity sends impulses to nerves throughout the body;
2 Those nerve firings result in muscle contractions;
3 Muscle contractions result in behaviors;
4 Perception sends updated info to the brain;
5 Go back to (1).

we see that steps (1) and (2) are importantly bound up with one another. The brain is still the central controller, but it's a central controller that is informed by more peripheral elements. But this puts an interesting spin on an objection to libertarianism. Recall that the libertarian maintains that human action is absolutely free and not determined. The obstacle to overcome is that the brain seems to be the controller of human action; since the brain is a physical object and determined by physical laws, human action is determined. But now the brain isn't the sole locus of activity generating human action. Instead, it's the whole body. So instead of accounting for how human behavior is independent of the brain, the libertarian story has to explain how human behavior is independent of the human body. We think there are ways to cope with this concern, but they'll take us too far afield for right now.

Side quest: But we can pick up this thread in a sidequest. G.E.M. Anscombe—and later, Ian Hacking[15]—developed the idea of "action under a description." To get the flavor, imagine you're making yourself a peanut butter and jelly sandwich. There are at least two ways to respond to the question, "what are you doing?" (i) You're making a PB&J and (ii) you're making lunch. If you're making it for a friend who broke her leg, you might also be (iii) helping your friend. Read the entry "Acting under a description" in *Wikipedia* and begin to sketch ideas for how that might help the weak-embodiment libertarian.

It also helps in filling out the details of Hume's classical compatibilism. Recall that Hume endorses psychological determinism: our mental states determine our actions. A further point for Hume is that all thoughts either (i) began as perception or (ii) are a remix of previous perceptions (like when you're imagining a flying goat). But with weak embodiment, we know that the body shapes our concepts, as with conceptual metaphor theory. (Jump back to Chapter 7 if you don't remember.) Psychological determinism takes on a new flavor when incorporating the body into perception, cognition, and desire. Perception informs *what* we think about, but the body's informing our conceptual repertoire informs *how* we think about it. So psychological determinism depends (in part) on our bodily condition. It's not just our minds that determine behavior. It's our bodies in conjunction with the mind that determines behavior.

12.10.2 Embodiment reframing questions

We saw above that taking the mind as embodied helps reframe questions in this space. Typically, the question is "are we free or determined?" and responses don't always consider the ways in which we're embodied.

They do to *some* extent, but it's mostly as a way of considering whether biological descriptions of human actions are sufficient to explain why we do what we do.

From a standpoint of strong embodiment, we're compelled to consider the role of the environment in pretty significant ways—not only in the context of action but also in the development of our habits. And the target of analysis shifts from thinking about the mind or brain in isolation to thinking about the mind or brain as it lives in our bodies in an environment. Beliefs, intentions, and desires aren't "in the head" as representation-heavy views contend. Rather, they come out in our bodily behaviors. Additionally, we might think of mental states as shorthand for how the world shows up for a person.

In particular, when we think about how cognition "extends" into the world, the stuff we rely on and the places we find ourselves are part of the cognitive system. If we ascribe responsibility or autonomy in virtue of mental states or other cognitive entities, then a whole lot of the world just came into the scope of thinking about responsibility. In other words, the sorts of cases where we thought we were interested in freedom of action might actually be cases of freedom of opportunity.

In short, when we consider the ways in which we're embodied, the traditional dichotomies of mind and body just don't work as well. In some ways, this is a breath of fresh air. We're biological organisms in addition to being things that think, and our conception of free will and autonomy should reflect that. But in other ways, this muddies the waters. Freedom and action are no longer a matter of hidden, occult entities. Instead, we're to take the environment and history into account. And putting this into a legal context? More philosophically sophisticated for sure, but so much cloudier in thinking about guilt and innocence.

Notes

1 Libertarianism in metaphysics is different from libertarianism in political philosophy. In metaphysics, it means what we said above: you make your choices freely. In political philosophy, it's about the role of the government in citizens' lives.

2 Parental lectures in our youth suggested we would be facing this dilemma a lot more than we actually did.

3 Suppose, in an act of random behavior, you channel your inner Jim Morrison and shout "ride the snake" to unsuspecting passers-by. When your friend asks you why you did it, you might shrug and say you just wanted to. That's it. Your wanting to is all the reason you need to perform some bit of arbitrary behavior.

4 Someone will of course say, "sure you have a choice—you could choose to be shot!" I suppose that's true. But if we took that seriously, then the police responding to the incident could reasonably ask, "why did you hand over your

wallet? You could have said, 'no.' That's on you." This is a counterintuitive situation. If you're robbed, it's the robber who is responsible for your missing wallet, not you.

5 For details, see "Homeownership, racial segregation, and policy solutions to racial wealth equity," from the Brookings Institute: https://www.brookings.edu/articles/homeownership-racial-segregation-and-policies-for-racial-wealth-equity/

6 This is the argument David Hume offers in *An Enquiry Concerning Human Understanding*.

7 Another example: you might wish you were the sort of person who likes jazz. You don't want to listen to jazz, but you have a desire to have a desire to listen to jazz. You might represent it as: I want x, where x is the desire to listen to jazz. These are **second-order desires**.

8 "C.R.E.A.M.": Cash Rules Everything Around Me. This is likely a reference to a song of the same name by the Wu-Tang Clan, released in 1994, in which Clan members Raekwon, Inspectah Deck, and Method Man describe the difficulties of growing up in poverty-stricken areas of New York, particularly Staten Island, and aspire to get rich.

9 There are some distinctions to be made between the concepts of agency and autonomy, but we're going to treat them as more or less synonymous.

10 The earliest a "No Fault Divorce" law was codified was 1969 in California. If your husband was emotionally or verbally (and even physically) abusive, it could be difficult to prove. Without No Fault Divorce, women were often unable to separate from their husbands.

11 Again, this isn't every case—some women, for example, might have breast implants after a mastectomy. Many people have many reasons, but this one is common enough to call out on its own. Further, this isn't good or bad. Some women may feel compelled to satisfy conventional norms of appearance. Other women may be happy satisfying conventional norms of appearance. This is a matter of debate in **third-wave feminism**.

12 For readers not familiar with American geography or history, North Carolina was a part of the Confederacy during the American Civil War. Many Africans and African-Americans were bought and sold there as well as enslaved on plantations. The legacy of slavery—as well as racist laws passed in the decades following the end of the Civil War—persisted through the 1960s into today.

13 In 1896, the US Supreme Court upheld the "separate but equal" doctrine in Plessy v. Ferguson: segregation was permissible as long as the facilities were separate but equal. This was overturned in 1954 in the case of Brown v. Board of Education. The point is that in 1960, segregation wasn't required and in fact was illegal.

14 Another footnote for unfamiliar readers: Virginia is another state in the American South. Its capital, Richmond, was the capital of the Confederacy.

15 See especially his book *The Social Construction of What?*.

13

ETHICS AND EMBODIMENT

13.1 Chapter overview

In your typical ethics course, three views are introduced: consequentialism, deontology, and virtue ethics. Thinking about ourselves as embodied introduces a set of new questions for each of these theories.

13.2 Introduction

If you're here for the embodiment, why should you care about ethics? What's the connection between ethics and embodiment? First, we are embodied organisms, and so a theory about how we ought to treat each other should reflect that. A moral theory that disregards embodiment is not a moral theory for embodied humans like us because it misses a crucial aspect of what it is to be human.

Another reason is to show that embodiment isn't just an issue for philosophy of mind or psychology. It connects with many areas of our lives. As we will see, thinking about ourselves as embodied can have significant consequences for how we think about ourselves and others.

Ethics is an *enormous* field. Normative ethics (sometimes called "ethical theory") asks questions like "what principles should govern my choices? What is valuable?" There's also **metaethics**, which considers questions like "what is it that makes moral statements true or false? Is goodness a property of the world, like mass?" Finally, **applied ethics** asks questions like "what does such-and-such moral theory advise us to do in *these* circumstances?" where "these circumstances" refer to a specific time and place. And within each of these divisions, there are further subdivisions.

DOI: 10.4324/9781003356622-16

In this chapter, we're going to focus on normative ethics. We're going to cover three major moral theories—consequentialism, deontology, and virtue ethics—and make some connections with theories of embodiment.

When we're looking at the impacts of theories of embodiment on our moral theories, we're going to do this in two ways. First, we're going to say, "given our moral theories, what can embodiment contribute to the conversations?" Here, we will take the moral theories as more or less settled and look at what questions embodiment considerations prompt. Second, we're going to say, "given our theories of embodiment, what kinds of moral issues are important?" This time, we'll develop our moral theory around our ideas of embodiment.

Remember in Chapter 6 when we talked about Neurath's Boat? Our worldviews are like boats we're building as we're sailing on them. In this chapter, we're going to "stand" on moral theory and ask questions about embodiment and then "stand" on embodiment and ask questions about moral theory.

13.3 Consequentialism

Imagine you find yourself faced with a choice. Your friend is going to fail a class and needs your help. They haven't been keeping up with the reading or the assignments, and they have 24 hours to complete an entire semester of work. They ask—no, they *beg*—you to share your work from when you took the class last year. If they fail this class, they'll lose their scholarship and have to drop out of school. They promise they've learned their lesson. Starting Day 1 of next semester, they'll be a model of organization and industry. You're torn about what to do.

On the one hand, giving your work to your friend could really help them. It'll help them pass the class and, more importantly, help them stay in school. Your friend failing out of college would have enormous negative effects. Besides (you think to yourself), it's a class that has nothing to do with your friend's major.

On the other hand, you might get caught, and then you're both sunk. Professors have all sorts of tools now to tell if a student has plagiarized or used another's work. You have no idea whether your friend's professor uses those kinds of tools. The chances you'll get caught are somewhere between 1% and 99%, but you have no idea what they are.

We'll leave it up to you to decide what to do, but there's something important to notice here. The kinds of considerations we're thinking through are what happens as a result of your choice. That is, we're looking at the *consequences* of your actions. A consequentialist argues that the most important consideration when thinking through moral issues is the consequences of your actions.

The basic intuition is that our actions have consequences and what matters are those outcomes: are people helped or harmed? This way of thinking has a kind of naturalness to it. We have good senses of what helps and what hurts and it's intuitively bad to hurt people (without *a* good reason).

But our actions have *loads* of consequences. Saying to your friend "no, sorry, I won't help you" moves air molecules, puts some carbon dioxide into the air, causes your friend to have a pit in their stomach, and so on. Which consequences are flagged as important gives rise to different kinds of consequentialism.

One theory focuses on pleasure and pain: right actions maximize pleasure and minimize pain. Another theory focuses on happiness and kinds of pleasures: right actions maximize happiness and minimize unhappiness, and maximizing happiness means pursuing intellectual pleasures over physical ones.

13.4 Deontology

Deontology is most strongly associated with Immanuel Kant. "Deon" means *duty*; deontology is the study of what our duties are. Duty, in this context, means what we are obligated to do, what we morally have to do (or not do).

To get a feel for this view, think about something you would never do, no matter what. There's no amount of money or cookies or fame anyone could offer you that would compel you to do this thing. It might be something incredibly violent, or maybe it would require betraying someone you love. Whatever that action is, you would never choose to do it, no matter how much it could benefit you.

This one might be a bit harder: what is an action that you must perform, no matter what? No matter how much money was offered to you to do something else, you must do this action. One candidate is returning what is borrowed: you must always return someone's property to them. Another might be telling the truth: you must always tell the truth.

This is the basic intuition behind deontological ethics: some actions are obligated—you morally must perform them. Other actions are forbidden—you may never perform them. If an action is obligated or forbidden, you're bound to do it (or not) no matter what the consequences might be.

The big question is: how do we figure out what our duties are? We'll be following Kant to answer this question.[1] In short, the answer is: autonomy. Usually, we are responsible for only those actions we choose to perform.[2] Our autonomy—our capacity to choose—is the basis for our assessments of responsibility and obligation.

Another way of putting this is to say that moral agents[3] are autonomous. If we fail to treat someone as autonomous, then we fail to treat them as a moral agent. So we are obligated to treat others in ways that respect their status as a moral agent. It's always and everywhere wrong to undermine a person's autonomy. This is a version of Kant's **categorical imperative**: treat people as ends in themselves and never as means. In other words: don't use people. When you manipulate someone or lie to them, you aren't letting them make choices for themselves. You're curating information so that they have one sort of response instead of another. You're not letting them choose how they'll react to the whole picture. Generally, any time you inhibit another person's ability to make their own choices—whether explicitly by making the choice for them or implicitly by manipulating them into making the choice you want them to make—you are infringing on their autonomy.

Otto's workbook: Consider again the predicament of your friend from the previous section: your friend begs you for your work from last semester, and you're conflicted about what to do. We're supposed to treat people as autonomous agents and not as things. What does that look like in this context? Should you give your friend your materials from last semester? Is it infringing on their autonomy to refrain from giving them your work?

13.5 Virtue ethics

This is an old tradition in ethics, stretching back to at least Plato, Aristotle, and Confucius. The core idea is that it's not outcomes or actions that are the primary focus of a moral theory. Instead, it is **character**. A person's character is what they're like: are they kind or mean? Funny or serious? Careless or careful? Our goal isn't to focus on *what we do* or the *outcomes* of what we do; we focus on *who we are*. We should do the best we can to become **virtuous** people.

Examples of virtues include compassion, bravery, and patience. They are qualities that make for a good life. Consider some religious traditions. From the Christian Scriptures, the story of the good Samaritan—a man who stops to help another who had been robbed and assaulted—demonstrates compassion. The Prophet's bravery is described in the Quran in many places. Job from the Hebrew Scriptures exemplifies patience and faith. A Buddhist koan tells of a farmer who met every turn of fortune with acceptance, never describing any event as good or bad; this farmer exemplifies wisdom.

One of the more famous accounts of virtue comes from **Aristotle.**[4] He describes virtue as being a kind of median state, often called the **Golden Mean,** with respect to how intensely a person feels their emotions. The goal of the virtuous person is to have the right sorts of responses to the right sorts of situations. Let's go through a few scenarios regarding anger.

- Suppose someone cuts you off in traffic, and you fly off the handle, tailgating them and following them to their home. In this case, you have gotten too angry. It's good to be a little angry in this scenario, but following a person to their home is going too far.
- Imagine your friend has just stolen your life's savings. You say "darn that Jerry!" and go about the rest of your day. Here, you're not angry enough. You should be very angry that your friend has taken everything from you.
- Suppose someone compliments your sense of style. Without an extensive backstory, it's wrong to get angry in this scenario.
- Imagine you're at a funeral and you've just learned that someone has stolen your identity. It's okay to be angry and excuse yourself to take care of the matter. It's not okay to jump up during the eulogy to shout "dammit! Someone stole my identity!"
- If you put laxatives in my brownies, it's wrong to get angry with anyone but you for that (again, absent an extensive backstory about a terrorist holding your family hostage and demanding you put laxatives in my brownies).

What these examples suggest is that being virtuous is a matter of experiencing your emotions to the right degree, in the right sorts of situations, and directed at the right people for the right reasons. Doing this requires **practical wisdom:** a kind of deep understanding of what the situation requires of you in the moment.[5] And when you're trying to figure out the best response, you can imagine what a virtuous person would do. For example, what would St. Oscar Romero, the Buddha, Rabbi Harold Kushner, Al-Ghazali, or Nelson Mandela advise? What would a wise grandparent say?

Otto's workbook: Consider one final time your friend who begs you for your old work. Think of a person you admire for their insight and wisdom. What would that person tell you to do?

13.6 Issues of embodiment in ethics

We've covered a few of the big theories in ethics. So how does embodiment relate to them? We're going to take this in two parts. First, we'll consider the ways that understanding minds as embodied informs our answers to questions posed by our current set of moral theories. Second, we'll consider how understanding minds as embodied changes the *kinds* of questions a moral theory should ask.

13.6.1 Consequentialism and embodiment

Consequentialism judges an action as right or wrong depending on the outcomes. **Jeremy Bentham**—a famous consequentialist—argued that the relevant moral question is *not* "does it think?" but rather "does it feel?" But how something feels can depend on the state of our bodies, both temporary and long-lasting. Consider a few examples:

- Congenital insensitivity to pain (CIP) is a rare genetic disorder in which pain receptors aren't functioning normally. People with CIP do not experience pain. This can cause serious problems since pain is a signal that something is wrong.[6] So if pain is bad and people with CIP don't feel physical pain, do we have to refrain from hurting them? If you meet someone with CIP, is it okay to hurt them since they won't feel it?
- Some people under the influence of controlled substances (under US law), like ecstasy (aka MDMA[7]) have a heightened sense of pleasure. Are our moral obligations to them different because they experience pleasure more acutely? If we could take such drugs with no negative side effects, would we be morally required to do so?

These questions revolve around the experiences of pleasure and pain we have in virtue of being embodied. But that's not the only way in which embodiment can matter for consequentialism. **John Stuart Mill** wrote,

> It is better to be a human being dissatisfied than a pig satisfied; better to be Socrates dissatisfied than a fool satisfied. And if the fool, or the pig, is of a different opinion, it is only because they only know their own side of the question.[8]

This raises some interesting questions about embodiment and our mental capacities. Both strong and weak embodiment argue that our cognitive processes are shaped by our bodies (albeit in different ways and to different extents). Socrates and the fool may have similar bodies in some morally superficial ways: they both have hearts, lungs, and so on. But when we start getting into more fine-grained mental capacities—like enjoying opera or sitcoms—our embodiment can differ in subtle ways. Recall that socialization is relevant to our embodiment. Whether we like opera or sitcoms can depend on our embodied upbringing, our affective response to opera or sitcoms. Mill's claims about Socrates and the fool assume that there is a common baseline by which to measure their satisfaction. The dissatisfaction of Socrates is "better" because Socrates is thinking more abstractly than the fool. Socrates can experience intellectual pleasures unavailable to the fool. But if socialization is part of embodiment and embodiment is relevant to our experiences of pleasure, why can't we just say that Socrates's pleasures are different, instead of better? Socrates and the fool had different socializations (let's suppose), so their embodied experiences will be different. What's the yardstick by which we can say that Socrates's pleasures are "higher" than those of the fool?

13.6.2 Deontology and embodiment

Kant's deontology values autonomy. But as we saw in the last chapter, autonomy isn't a simple concept and certainly isn't independent of our embodiment. In this context, the question to ask is: does being embodied affect our autonomy? That is: does being embodied affect how we are able to legislate the moral law to ourselves? (Remember "autonomy" comes from the Greek "auto" meaning *self* and "nomos" meaning *law*.)

If you think about the mind as separate from the body, then our embodiment doesn't make much of a difference. No matter whether you're you or your consciousness is uploaded to a machine, your autonomy is unaffected. Your ability to *act* on your choices can be affected: if your mind is uploaded to a computer, you may not have a voice to tell the truth. But your ability to choose is not.

Now Kant in his *Critique of Pure Reason* (and elsewhere) says,

> ... the action must be possible under natural conditions if the ought is directed to it; but these natural conditions do not concern the determination of the power of choice itself, but only its effect and result in appearance
>
> *(A548/B576)*

The part of the sentence before the semicolon[9] is sometimes referred to as the "**ought implies can**" principle: if you ought to do something, that implies you can do that thing. The **contrapositive** (which is logically equivalent to the original statement) is: if you *can't* do something, you *are not obligated* to do that something. Or what amounts to the same: if something is impossible, then you're not obligated to do it.

Consider then that what we're able to do is informed by our embodiment. This can happen in some superficial ways: if you have a sore throat and can't talk, then you're not obligated to tell the truth under those conditions.[10] But we can consider some deeper cases: someone with a disability might not be able to engage in some behaviors available to people without disabilities. Are there differences in moral obligations between people with and without disabilities? Furthermore, neurotypical and neurodiverse people can vary in what they are able to do. Are there different moral obligations for these groups? Once we start pointing out these differences in bodies, we lose one of the big advantages of a deontological theory: identifying objective rules for right and wrong action. But you get to make a decision: does that mean we accept the loss of objective rules or do we disregard embodiment as important for morality?

13.6.3 Virtue theory and embodiment

There's a clear sense in which embodiment is relevant to virtues. In order to possess and exercise a virtue, you have to have the right emotional response to a situation. If you are too angry or insufficiently angry, then you're not enacting the virtue. You're coming close, but not hitting the mark. Since emotions are part of our embodiment and emotions are relevant to virtues, embodiment is relevant to virtues. But can we do more than this? Here's where we're going to experience some more *aporia*. But first, a little background information…

There's a line of research from social psychology starting in the 1950s that looks at the effects of the environment and conformity pressures on decision making. In 1951, psychologist Solomon Asch published a paper looking at the effects of group pressure on judgments. Long story short: some participants went along with the crowd to say one line was longer than another when that was very obviously not the case. One of Asch's students, Stanley Milgram, published a remarkable and upsetting study in 1963. Ordinary folks showed that they were willing to shock unknown subjects at dangerously high voltages if the experimenter asked them to do so, even when the subject pleaded for the experiment to be stopped. How did they know the voltage was high? Because the device used in the experiment was labeled "Danger: Severe Shock."[11] In 1973, John Darley and Daniel Batson published their famous Good Samaritan study. Again, to make a long story short, seminarians were more likely to help someone in need only when they had the time to do so. And there have been *countless* studies looking at the effects of the social environment on judgment and action. The results? Not good: we often think we're making decisions and choices independently, but they're often the result of forces outside our control.

In the early 2000s, philosophers like Gilbert Harman and John Doris introduced this psychology literature into moral philosophy. They argued that whether we perform a virtuous action isn't a result of character but rather of the situation in which we find ourselves. This cluster of positions is known as **situationism**. There are a few ways of developing the main idea, but it says, roughly, that our idea of someone's character as a stable and long-lasting feature of their personality isn't as important when evaluating someone's actions or judgments as we take it to be. Your good actions (but also your bad ones) aren't entirely attributable to you.[12]

Where this takes an interesting turn is in considering the extended mind (and similar views under the label of "strong embodiment"). The environment, or at least parts of it, is part of the cognitive system. The line between mind and world is fuzzier. So what does that mean for our ideas about character and virtue? Let's consider two cases.

First, we might endorse Clark and Chalmers's extended mind, thinking of specific items in the environment as part of the cognitive system. Suppose you promise a friend that you'll pick them up at the airport. You schedule an alarm on your phone so you don't forget. Now imagine that you're out and about on the day you're to pick them up. Your phone dies, but you don't notice. It's not until several hours after the scheduled pick-up time that it hits you: you were supposed to be at the airport hours ago. You pull your phone from your pocket to see that it's dead. You race home to plug in your phone and see that you have literally dozens of missed calls and texts from your friend, who is angry that you've broken your promise. You call your friend, who ended up taking a taxi home, and explain that it wasn't your fault. You had the reminder set on your phone, but then your phone died. Your friend, a student of philosophy, replies that the phone is part of your extended cognitive system. You offloaded a task onto the phone. But it doesn't make a difference if the information is located in your frontal lobe or your phone: you are blameworthy all the same. You failed to take the necessary steps to ensure that your phone was in working order. Your friend draws an analogy: imagine you imbibed too much alcohol and forgot to pick them up. You'd certainly be blameworthy. But failing to make sure your phone is charged is no different: you engaged in some actions that resulted in your cognitive system not being in working order. Therefore, you are responsible for failing to fulfill your promise.

Otto's workbook: What do you think of your friend's argument?

Once we start thinking of external objects as part of the cognitive system, assessing responsibility becomes trickier for virtue theories. This is because virtue theories assess the person's character. If your cognitive system extends outside your body, then there's a case to be made that your moral character likewise extends.[13] If your moral character extends outside your body, then where you are and what you have ready to hand are part of the assessment of your actions and choices. Is your friend right? Is not making sure your phone is fully charged like imbibing too much alcohol? You may agree or disagree, but that's possible because of how we're thinking about the extended mind.

Now let's consider the second case. You might remember the concept of an *Umwelt* from the chapter on strong embodiment (Chapter 9). An *Umwelt* is your niche—how the world shows up for you. We mentioned that cultural and social influences inform the construction of your niche. If that's right, then the moral world is also part of your *Umwelt*. With that connection, a lot of interesting questions and problems crop up. For example, suppose some action doesn't show up for you as wrong—does that mean it's okay? How do we settle moral differences across *Umwelten*?

Otto's workbook: How can you settle moral differences across cultures? Is it even possible?

Because virtue theory has elements of embodiment baked into it, we're going to use consequentialism and deontology as our comparisons to an embodiment-first ethics.

13.7 Embodiment and reframing questions in ethics

Let's take embodiment as given and see what sorts of moral issues we generate from there. We'll make our way in by employing a few of the concepts from the chapter on strong embodiment.

13.7.1 Objective, intersubjective, and subjective

Remember that for the strong embodiment theorist, we engage in sensemaking. We construct the meaningfulness of the world for ourselves.

And what's meaningful evokes emotional reactions. Our moral lives revolve around what is meaningful for us.

What are some of the things that are meaningful for us? The first thing to notice is that *lots* of people have common things that are meaningful. Sure, there will be exceptions, but those are the *exceptions*, not the rule. What are some of these things? First, caring for one's offspring. For most parents, their kids are meaningful to them and for them. For instance, we would recoil in horror if a parent were to casually mention that they had a second child in case the first one ever needed an organ transplant.

> **Otto's workbook**: A deontologist would agree that having a second child for spare parts is bad. The view we're exploring now says it's bad because children are meaningful to their parents. What would be the deontologist's explanation? Do you find one view more persuasive than the other?

Something else widespread that people find meaningful is their own well-being. How you're doing is important to *you* (and to other people too, but we're talking about you right now).[14] We are not indifferent to our lives and the ways they unfold. Your life is *yours* and important to you for that reason. Note that how we experience the importance of our own well-being will differ from one culture to another. For example, Americans find high self-esteem to be very important, while the Japanese do not.[15] This doesn't mean that Japanese people are depressed or that they don't care about themselves. Rather, Japanese (and most collectivist cultures) conceptualize the self as overlapping with others.[16] We find this same point again in the concept of a "midlife crisis." This is experienced in American culture as a kind of existential crisis about the significance of one's life.[17] This is an expression of the meaningfulness of one's life to oneself.

> **Otto's workbook**: What are some other things that you think are meaningful for a significant population of people? It doesn't have to be the majority of humanity. Think also about your culture or social group.

We want to stress this point because it mirrors one that we saw in Chapter 9 about sensorimotor contingencies. Just as there are many overlaps in individuals' perceptual systems, there are many overlaps in what individuals find meaningful. It is *not* **subjective**: there are commonalities we can observe and reflect on. Instead, what we find meaningful is often

intersubjective. Meaningfulness isn't just located in my head; nor is it an agent-independent property of the world. It is a property that comes out of historical and current interpersonal interactions. It's not what *I* find meaningful; it's what *you and I* find meaningful. This takes place at small scales with just a handful of people and also at large scales with entire populations (neighborhoods, cities, cultures, etc.).

But also, notice that meaningfulness isn't **objective** either: it's not a property of a mind-independent world, definable apart from our own needs and interests.[18] Nothing is meaningful in itself. In this way, meaningfulness isn't like size or shape. Consequentialism values outcomes; those are meaningful in virtue of the amount of happiness or harm they put into the world. Happiness and harm depend on us (after all, we're the ones who are happy or harmed), but their meaningfulness doesn't necessarily depend on us. Deontology values duties; those are meaningful because they're grounded in the concept of autonomy. And while *we* are the ones who are autonomous, the meaningfulness of autonomy doesn't necessarily depend on us. If we take sense-making as our starting point, then our moral theories begin with our being in the world and being with each other. Meaningfulness is grounded in *us*.

Why does this matter? It matters for how we understand moral decisions. For objective theories, it can happen that the right action is already determined by the theory, and we need to figure out what it is. If you are thinking about shoplifting a candy bar, that will cause some amount of pleasure and pain. Your job as a moral agent is to consider how much pleasure and pain it causes and then act accordingly. The rule for acting is settled without your input. But if we have an intersubjective view, then rules for acting are settled *with* our input. It's entirely possible that, for some decisions, there is no rule or precedent to follow. In these cases, there's little to fall back on for discerning which action is right.

13.7.2 Emotion and sense-making

Now we saw that what is meaningful also elicits emotional responses and that sense-making is about constructing what's meaningful. This has two implications. First, let's think about decision-making. For all the views we saw above, reason played a primary role. The consequentialist says to figure out the consequences; deontology says reason is our guide to figuring out our obligations. Virtue ethics is different. A central part of being virtuous is cultivating the right emotions. On the strong embodiment view, emotions are inseparable from sense-making. When something is meaningful for us—whether good or bad—it evokes emotions in us. Emotions are worked into how we understand and perceive the world. Reason and emotion on this account *can't* be split. When we choose an action, that choice is informed by a multitude of capacities that are tangled up together: reason, emotion, sense-making, and affordance pick-up, to name just a few. The advice to "think rationally" is nonsense on this view, since reason is bound up with emotion.

So why is that significant? One important feature is that it highlights how people see the world as part of the decision-making. The other moral frameworks introduced in this chapter presume that there is a mind-independent world about which we reason. The meaningfulness of *anything* is imposed on it by us.[19] This is a two-step process: make sure your beliefs correspond to the world and then evaluate an action according to some moral framework, which specifies what has value.

On the strong-embodiment view, meaning is co-constructed; it is intersubjective. The idea of a mind-independent world onto which we impose values just doesn't make sense here. A better metaphor, as compared to matching and imposing, is perceiving and recognizing. We perceive and recognize meaning and value in the world, which guide our choices. This is a one-step process. So when we're making a decision, we're recognizing what we ought to do in the world. The cool difference here is in how we think about the engine behind our choices: is it our beliefs and desires? Or is it the world? Is it *me* who is the ground of my choices? Or is it *something much bigger but still part of me?*

The second implication is interacting with others. **Participatory sense-making** is a kind of sense-making that we do with others. Of course, how we make sense of things is a product of our culture, our society, our upbringing, and many others besides. *Participatory* sense-making makes the role of the other explicit in our interactions. It's a kind of coordination among individuals as a part of sense-making.

For example, imagine two people, Judith and Tamar. Judith says something that hurts Tamar's feelings; however, Judith didn't think she said anything hurtful to Tamar. Now, suppose Tamar shares her hurt feelings. Together, Judith and Tamar can make sense of the interaction. Notice that there are three possibilities: (a) Judith sees that her remark was hurtful and apologizes to Tamar; (b) Tamar realizes she misunderstood Judith and no longer feels hurt; and (c) neither moves but rather doubles down on the initial beliefs and feelings. In any of these cases, Judith and Tamar make sense of the original interaction with each other. When either Judith or Tamar changes their beliefs, their initial understandings shift to align with those of the other. In case (c), instead of getting in sync, they get into "anti-sync." If syncing is Judith and Tamar zigging and zagging together, anti-syncing is when Judith zigs and Tamar zags. They've still coordinated with one another, but each person's movements are the opposite of the other.

13.7.3 Umwelt, *intentionality, and empathy*

Remember that your *Umwelt* is the environment as it shows up for you, chock full of meaning and value. Things in your *Umwelt* show up with an emotional valence: apples and oranges show up as edible and safe; growling dogs show up as threatening. We also noted that one's *Umwelt* is shaped by social and cultural events and processes. What appears safe to one social group appears dangerous to another.

Also, recall that intentionality is a kind of "gearing into" the world. Our beliefs and desires about the world are directed toward the world and not internal representations. Our mental states and experiences are about how we're engaged with the world.

You are engaged with the coffee cup with respect to how you can interact with it and what you can do with it. But we don't engage with other people in the same way that we engage with coffee mugs: we *use* coffee mugs, but we don't (or at least shouldn't) use people. So how are we engaged with other people?

There's one line of thinking in strong embodiment that says **empathy** is how we are engaged with others. Evan Thompson, in his paper "Empathy and Consciousness," argues that consciousness is intersubjectively constituted. In other words, there is no consciousness without other people. How does this work? Whenever you look at something, you only see one aspect of the thing's profile. As you look at your phone, you have a sense that there's another side, even though you can't see it. What is this sense? Where does it come from? Thompson (following Husserl) argues that it comes from correlates of the possible perceptions of other people. In other words, you have a sense that your phone has a back you can't see because your consciousness is structured in such a way that you automatically "know" what other people's perspectives look like.[20]

This means that our perception of the world and the sense of an object's wholeness are constituted by your perception and what things would look like from others' points of view. But what things look like from other points of view is another way of talking about empathy! Our perception of the world has empathy built into it. We couldn't have perceptual experiences without empathy.

Let's pull the big ideas together:

1 Empathy is built into how we perceive and experience the world;
2 Our experiences of the world are intersubjective;
3 Therefore, empathy is built into intersubjectivity.

In relating to others, we're always already exercising empathy. You cannot fail to exercise empathy in relating to others. This has significant moral implications. Experiences of the world and relating to others are soaked with emotion and meaning. How we experience the world and each other is an emotional process that's full of meaning. While we can't experience the world from others' perspectives, we can empathize with others. We can imagine anger or happiness as part of different experiences, even if we have never undergone those experiences.

For example, we (AK and CL) are both middle-aged, white men—about as vanilla as it gets. We have never, nor could we ever, experience racism or sexism as other people have. Even so, we are able to empathize with those who have experienced discrimination. We make sense of such experiences in terms of the ideas and experiences that we have had.

If my (CL) friend tries to communicate to me her frustration and anger with being told, "you got that job only because you're a woman," my sense-making capacities enable me to correlate that with experiences that I have had, like failures to recognize my talents and diminishings of my accomplishments.

In principle, then, others' experiences are empathizable to some degree because of the nature of our consciousness. Just as I have a sense that the phone has a backside because of others' perspectives, I have a sense of others' experiences because I can take up others' perspectives (to some degree).

13.7.4 Differences between embodiment-first ethics and traditional approaches

You may have noticed some differences in the kinds of questions being asked in Section 13.7 as opposed to Section 13.6. Consequentialism asks "what action maximizes some good outcome?" An embodiment-first approach to ethics asks "how do we navigate this dilemma?" This is because, at least partly, the background metaphysics for some traditional views is more or less set (or is neutral regarding the claims of the moral theory). In other words, as long as you are a rational agent, it doesn't matter to consequentialism if you are an identity theorist or a functionalist. Similarly with deontology: as long as you're a rational agent, the background metaphysics of mind don't matter.[21]

On embodiment-first views, it *does* matter how we conceive of being a rational agent. We saw in the last section that empathy is part of the structure of consciousness on some views of embodiment, and we got there through consideration of intersubjectivity and, by extension, embodiment. The moral considerations we develop through this approach are not neutral with respect to the nature of the agent.

It may turn out that an embodiment-first ethics can offer a decision procedure like consequentialism or some strands of deontology.[22] Even if it can, that's not what's most interesting about an embodiment-first approach.

This sort of approach takes people and their environments as a given and then asks what we owe to others from there. We're carving up the boundaries of agents differently: you aren't your brain or even just your body. You are a rational entity whose activities are spread out over body and world. That is, *given* that we're embodied and situated in social and cultural networks, how are we to act? What should one do? Consider participatory sense-making. There are people with morally reprehensible views with whom you might need to make sense of something. Do we *negotiate* meanings with them? Ideally, you would "pull" them from the morally worrisome views to the morally acceptable ones; but that treats participatory sense-making as a one-way street, which isn't really *participatory*.

13.8 Care ethics

Care ethics is similar to virtue ethics in that the details of particular cases are crucial. All moral judgments are context-sensitive. It is dissimilar to virtue ethics in the sense that the aim is one of care, and care is fundamentally about relationships.[23] We mention care ethics as a theoretical framework separate from the others because it builds embodiment into the ground level of the theory. Care ethics takes embodied and situated individuals as its starting point for moral reflection. However, it's not typically counted among the "Big 3" of moral frameworks, which is another reason why we're setting it apart from the others.[24]

The origins of care ethics can be traced to the work of psychologist **Carol Gilligan**, who challenged the dominating moral development framework of **Lawrence Kohlberg**. Gilligan noticed that girls and women tended to score lower than men on Kohlberg's scale of moral development. In her work, she uncovered that girls and women placed a higher premium on relationships than abstract moral principles. Those relationships revolved around ideas of care. One reason why the girls and women described care as an important moral dimension is that they are often socialized into caring roles as parents and caretakers. Women are often expected to be "naturally" caring, in part because of cisgendered women's role as biological mothers.

Care is difficult to define, but your everyday understanding of it is probably just fine for our purposes. Paradigm examples of care are the ways in which we care about our friends and family. You show care for your friends by spending time with them, listening to them, and helping them through tough times. Parents show care for children by feeding and clothing them, as well as being interested in their hobbies and disciplining them.

Virginia Held, one prominent care ethicist, describes care in terms of motives, feelings, and behaviors.[25] To be a caring person, you have to *actually* be engaged in relationships of care. It's not enough to have caring motives or caring emotions. The actual engagement is important because care is a relation among persons. Whenever we enact care, we do it *for* someone. You care for your friends; parents care for their children. You can care for yourself! But care is always about someone involving at least two people. Additionally, care is a two-way street. To care about your friend, your friend needs to care about you. The care in each direction might look different: the way parents care for children is different from how children care for parents. But the caring person will look to make their existing relationships ones of care.

One of the features of care ethics that relates to this book is that care ethics begins from a place of embodiment and situatedness. All of us are embodied and found in a set of relationships within a social and cultural context. It is from here that we begin thinking about the concept of care and what an ethics of care entails. For example, suppose you're in charge of getting food for a birthday party that will be attended by some of your friends. You're not sure of everyone's dietary needs, but you know that some of your friends will require halal foods and others will need gluten-free foods. Enacting care in this instance is making sure that those friends have things they can eat. Notice that this is attending to the embodied and cultural dimensions of your friends.

Care ethics emphasizes that caring relationships are always with embodied people who are situated in places. It begins with the messiness of our everyday lives. Sometimes, the embodied dimension of enacting care means attending to someone's biological needs. Other times, the embodied dimension of enacting care defines some of our caring relationships. Mothers have a distinct caring relationship with their children because they gave birth to them. Romantic and sexual relationships are sometimes distinguished from other close relationships in virtue of the physical intimacy of the partners. Such physical intimacy informs what care looks like in some cases.

Lastly, care ethics reflects facts about embodiment with respect to recognizing limits of care. Every last one of us has limits that vary from day to day. Parents can experience burnout from caring for their children. Parents bump up against their limits. Care in these times is going to look different from care at other times because the parents don't have the physical or mental ability to show the same sort of care.

13.9 Conclusion

The big takeaway from this chapter is that embodiment matters for how we think about our responsibilities to others and the wider world. If you're a disembodiment sort of person, then the character of the environment—that is, your *Umwelt*—is going to be less obviously relevant to deliberating about what to do or how to hold people accountable. Emotions and making sense of the world are not on the horizon of disembodied moral thinkers. They could be, but it's not obvious in the way that they are for strong embodiment theorists.

Does this mean that to be moral, you have to believe that strong embodiment is the right view of the mind? No, but strong embodiment does highlight features of our moral lives that are important to reflect on. Independent of whether you think that minds are embodied, it's still worthwhile to consider the role of empathy and sense-making in moral reflection. This takes us back to Section 6.5, where we described possible information about a theory of the mind in terms of signal and noise: when we're considering how we are to treat others, what's relevant and what's not?

Notes

1 Kant is a very influential philosopher in the Western tradition. As you might imagine, there are a lot of interpretations of Kant and Kantian ethics. We think our presentation is relatively uncontroversial, but some might disagree.
2 This isn't always the case. Parents can be responsible for their children's behaviors or military officers can be responsible for the behaviors of their subordinates.
3 There are also "moral patients": individuals (human and non-human) who are incapable of making choices but nonetheless deserve moral consideration, like a baby or someone in a coma.
4 There are other sorts of virtue ethics. For instance, David Hume develops an ethics of virtue.
5 You might be thinking, "wow, this moral theory is incredibly vague." You're not wrong. It doesn't offer precise guidance like consequentialism or deontology. This is, in part, because virtue theories tend to focus on the details of particular situations. There are some rules of thumb that apply across a lot of scenarios, but how you should respond is always going to be context-specific.
6 These folks can get infections, break bones, undergo damage to the cornea, and they don't know it. As you might imagine, this is a very bad thing.
7 MDMA = 3,4-Methylenedioxymethamphetamine
8 You can find a copy at *Project Gutenberg*: https://www.gutenberg.org/files/11224/11224-h/11224-h.htm
9 The part after the semicolon expresses that our power to choose is independent of the context of action.
10 Someone might respond that the ought-implies-can principle is to be understood under normal circumstances: normally you don't have laryngitis, so you're still obligated to tell the truth even if you can't do it right now. If you are inclined this way, ask yourself this: how would you begin spelling out "normal" conditions that don't refer to what's normal?
11 All the subjects of the experiment were later debriefed and told that they didn't actually hurt anyone.
12 Situationism was later extended into epistemology: our judgments and beliefs aren't entirely up to us but are rather the product of our upbringing and situation.

13 Or if not "extends", at least complicates the picture significantly.
14 When someone is indifferent to their own well-being, Western mental health professionals often take this as a sign of clinical depression. This is one of the exceptions to people finding their own well-being meaningful.
15 Heine, S. J., Lehman, D. R., Markus, H. R. & Kitayama, S. (1999). "Is there a universal need for positive self-regard?" *Psychological Review*, 106 (4), 766–794.
16 Markus, H. & Kitayama, S. (1991). "Culture and the self: Implications for cognition, emotion, and motivation," *Psychological Review*, 98 (2), 224–253.
17 Interestingly, this phenomenon doesn't show up in many East Asian cultures: for details see the essays in *Welcome to Middle Age! (And Other Cultural Fictions)*, edited by Richard Shweder (Chicago: University of Chicago Press, 1998).
18 There is one view in metaethics called *moral realism*, which says that moral properties are real and exist in the world. If you're going to adopt an intersubjective view of meaningfulness, does that mean you *can't* be a moral realist? A lot depends on the details here. If "realism" means *existing independently of our own needs and interests*, then you probably can't have an intersubjective view of meaningfulness and be a moral realist. But if you think about moral properties as being more like *social* properties, then yes you can probably have both. For example, *being a citizen* is a social property; it is a property only because there are nations and people to define them. If *being meaningful* is a property like *being a citizen*, then you can both have an intersubjective take on moral properties and be a moral realist.
19 This relates to an argument attributed to **David Hume** in *A Treatise of Human Nature* (book 3, part 1, section 1): the is-ought gap. In short, how things *are* in the world doesn't tell you how things *ought to be*. That is, you can't go from a description of something and from that alone figure out what should be done.
20 Why? If it's not other people, then the sense comes from your own possible perceptions of the object. It's something like this: you have a sense that your phone has a backside because you could move in such a way as to see the backside of the phone. This doesn't work. Your experience of the object is constituted by possible, but *not actual*, perceptions. The difficulty is how to explain our experience of a single object in terms of real and possible perceptions.
21 One exception to this is eliminativism: eliminating talk about mental states and instead appealing to brain states.
22 Kant, in *Groundwork for the Metaphysics of Morals*, presents one version of his Categorical Imperative as: don't act on a rule that couldn't be universalized. As an example, lying can't be universalized. For lying to succeed, the hearer has to think you're telling the truth. But lying in this case is universal, and no hearer would think you're telling the truth. Therefore, in a world where everyone lies, no one could ever successfully lie. Lying isn't a rule that could be universalized.
23 Virtues aren't necessarily about relationships. I might need another person in order to exercise charity, but I can still be a charitable person without enacting it.
24 Many introductory ethics textbooks don't discuss care ethics at all, which we think is too bad.
25 See in particular her 2006 book *The Ethics of Care: Personal, Political, and Global*.

14

TECHNOLOGY AND EMBODIMENT

14.1 Chapter overview

This chapter explores how our relationship with technology can be understood through the lens of embodied and extended cognition. We'll see that our devices aren't just tools we use, but can become integral parts of our cognitive processes, raising important questions about the nature of mind and our interactions with the world. We'll also delve into the implications of increasingly sophisticated and agentive technologies for how we think and act.

14.2 Socrates contra EM

In Plato's *Phaedrus*, Socrates famously expressed apprehension toward an emerging technology that extended cognition: writing. If we wrote things down, he cautioned, we wouldn't really know things anymore arguing that reliance on external written characters would diminish the use of memory, leading to forgetfulness in learners' souls:

> It [writing] will introduce forgetfulness into the soul of those who learn it: they will not practice using their memory because they will put their trust in writing, which is external and depends on signs that belong to others, instead of trying to remember from the inside, completely on their own...you have not discovered a potion for remembering [via the invention of writing] but for reminding, you provide your students with the appearance of wisdom, not with its reality.
>
> *(Phaedrus, 275)*

DOI: 10.4324/9781003356622-17

In ancient Greece (as well as many other cultures), knowledge was preserved and transmitted "in the head," through memorization and the spoken word–the oral tradition.[1] He warned that if we started writing things down (on stone tablets or papyrus), knowledge would leave our heads and dumb us down. Writing would merely provide the *appearance* of wisdom, as individuals would trust external signs instead of remembering for themselves.

It's unlikely Socrates was a proponent of EM; perhaps if he were, he might not have been as worried about our adoption and development of writing technologies. Much to his dismay, writing persists, as do many forms of knowledge representing knowledge *outside* of us (e.g., audio and video recordings).

Socrates' concern echoes in contemporary debates surrounding our relationship with technology–namely, electronic devices and online services. Just as Socrates feared the consequences of shifting from an internal to an external means of knowledge storage, many today voice similar anxieties about our dependence on smartphones, laptops, and the cloud. We increasingly store vast amounts of information externally, raising the question of whether this reliance diminishes our cognitive capacities or extends them.

But if we adopt EM, perhaps Socrates's anxieties, as well as our own, might be reframed. Rather than viewing writing or modern digital technologies as external threats to our cognitive faculties, we might consider them potential extensions of these faculties. As Clark and Chalmers remind us, the boundaries of the mind are not confined to the skull. As we've seen, under EM, these technologies are not just "useful tools" or entertainment–they are *literally* aspects of the mind, given our reliable coupling to them.

Side quest: What, if any, are the differences between Socrates' worry–moving from the oral to a written tradition–and our modern day 'tech' worry–an increasing dependence on electronic devices and online services? What (if any) are the differences between these two worries? Does reliance on external forms of knowledge diminish our cognitive capacities or extend them? Why? And, most importantly, why does this matter?

In what follows, we explore the notion that technology, far from being merely a set of external tools, can become deeply intertwined with our minds, as proposed by EM. But to get to the good stuff on this topic, we must move beyond simplistic reactions to technology, whether uncritical enthusiasm or dystopian pronouncements, and instead focus on specific phenomena (rather than a strawman-ish target like "technology"). We'll employ the philosophical frameworks developed throughout this book to achieve a more coherent understanding of the relationship between software products, services, electronic devices, and the mind. Our point here is to act as a springboard–to spark further examination of important topics in our everyday lives. In taking you through these problem spaces, we hope to guide more helpful, impactful, and novel applications of EM into more clearly scoped and less "noisy" areas of discussion often found when important philosophical issues butt up against significant changes in our lives.

14.3 Topics

> ... 'I' am a mind that spills far beyond this body along countless contingent lines of action, interaction and comprehension...my phone [for example] becomes a kind of intellectual prosthesis that not only enables but also *enacts* aspects of cognition. Take it away and I am altered in non-trivial ways. Install new apps, unveil new features, and I am non-trivially augmented. And I am by definition unaware of many of the most significant aspects of this augmentation until absence or alteration forces me to confront them.[2]

At this point in the book, it's easy for us to "get our heads around" the idea that being reliably coupled to objects like notebooks and chalkboards makes them constitutive parts of cognition (cf. reliable coupling and the parity principle). But in today's world, a significant portion of the population is reliably coupled to a wide array of electronic devices. According to EM, these devices are not simply useful aids but are part of our mind. As Clark argued, the smartphone, for most of us, functions as an already integrated component of our cognitive apparatus.[3] While this claim is interesting and probably true, it requires further exploration to have real-world implications. In our view, it's one thing for philosophy to show how concepts relate to things in the world, but it's another—arguably more important—task to take abstract relationships and try to tie them to concrete solutions or implications.

14.3.1 Where does the mind end and "technology" begin?

Consider how often we rely on our smartphones for information that would have previously required memorization or physical reference materials. This reliable access to information is a crucial criterion for extended cognition. According to the parity principle, if a part of the world functions as a process which, were it done in the head, we would have no hesitation in recognizing it as part of the cognitive process, then that part of the world is part of the cognitive process. So for many of us, the smartphone, with its capacity for information storage, navigation, communication, and even computational tasks, fulfills this functional role.

So when we say that "the iPhone is part of my mind already," the claim may be true, but it is too vague. We need to understand why and how the iPhone is part of my mind, that is, in virtue of which properties the iPhone has. This is where we need to look at which *product(s)* correlate with those properties.

We have to move beyond the high-level neo-functionalist argument that states, "I am reliably coupled to object Y, Y functions in the same way it would inside my head, therefore Y is part of my mind." Electronic objects possess a more complex and dynamic existence than static tools like Otto's notebook. When we broadly refer to "tech" or "electronics," we often lack the necessary precision for a nuanced philosophical analysis.

Consider the iPhone. As mere hardware, the physical device itself, is not particularly effective as an extension of our mind in all respects. A physical notepad might be more suitable for rapidly jotting down fleeting thoughts. What truly holds significance is that the iPhone is a reliable hardware platform that *realizes* software, and it is the interplay between the device and its software that performs functions extending our cognitive capacities. This distinction is not merely semantic. To adequately address crucial issues such as responsibility and the consequences of system failure, we must identify precisely what *realizes* the cognitive functions within the extended system.

14.3.2 Smartphone ontology

When we say "electronic device," we usually mean hardware *and* software. An iPhone qua hardware is useless as "part of my mind." I could maybe attach sticky notes to the phone, or carve a note into its sides, and carry it around with me, but a notepad of the same size would be a far better piece of hardware to extend my mind. But the iPhone qua hardware is certainly not what we have in mind, nor is it what Clark and Chalmers are after. What matters here is that the iPhone serves as a reliable piece of hardware that *realizes* software, and *in concert*, the electronic device realizes functions that extend my mind. This is not merely a pedantic point; it's critical to pinpoint what realizes the cognitive functions, otherwise our implications fall flat (e.g., we won't know who or what to examine or critique, nor will we know what's responsible if there are issues with my reliable coupling, information retrieval, etc.). But this is where things start to get weird.

For starters, these objects have a more complex existence than the kinds of "static hardware" we've talked about so far, like notebooks and chalkboards. Unfortunately, most conversations about "tech" or electronics are too vague to be helpful; whatever objects they're talking about tend to lack any meaningful (or actionable) precision. So let's try to be as specific as we can. It's more helpful to speak in terms of *products*. While this still is a pretty wide notion, it forces us to point to more concrete particular things than "technology." There are hardware products (things that take up obvious physical space) like iPhones, laptops, or keyboards, and there are software products (software applications, programs, or systems designed to solve specific problems or fulfill particular needs for a user base) like Google Chrome, MacOS, or Minecraft.

The iPhone qua hardware (hiPhone for short) enjoys a pretty obvious, observable existence. In philosophy, this speaks to its *ontological* status—*how* or *what it means* for the object to exist. It's no mystery where my hiPhone is; it's right where I put it last, on the shelf next to my desk. But where is the rest of it? Where is the iPhone qua electronic device? More importantly, *where* is the software?

This question is important for us because we should at least know where an object is if we're to be reliably coupled to it. This question doesn't come up with other kinds of objects: my notebook is confined to a finite space, and doesn't really "surprise" me and/or change its functions without my knowing; it doesn't exactly "shut off" in the same way electronic devices do (like if my iPhone "bricks" and stops working, turning back into a hiPhone).

Let's call my iPhone qua electronic device the ediPhone. The ediPhone's utility in extending my mind comes in virtue of its realizing the right kinds of software for me. I know that I can pull up the relevant app (e.g., Notes, Docs, Keep, etc.) and find all the information I put in there. This is where the ediPhone far exceeds Otto's notebook in terms of its ability to extend my mind: it contains a *lot* of information for me that I can reliably surface, modify, etc., serving as a superpowered form of my outside memory–that is, of course, provided the ediPhone works in a stable, reliable way.

Unfortunately, as most of us know from experience, electronic devices don't always work in a stable, reliable way, especially when compared to most static objects.[4] And when they don't work, my mind is "shut off." It's almost like having some kind of neural ablation. Memory loss here becomes more than something that happens to my hard drive; it's something that happens to my mind as well.

These are just some of the "ontological struggles" inherent in our reliance on such dynamic systems, particularly the software component. If Otto's consistently used notebook were to suddenly become blank due to damage, it would represent a significant disruption to his cognitive system—like a service interruption in a digital system. Similarly, if the notebook's handwriting style inexplicably changed or the pages began turning on their own, it would represent a fundamental alteration to the interface—akin to an interface change on a screen. These are not trivial occurrences; if we accept these systems as constitutive parts of our extended cognitive apparatus, then outages and interface changes bear resemblance to neural ablations and alterations in our internal cognitive processing.

This observation leads to a critical ethical question: if we are reliably coupled to a system that is characterized by constant updates and modifications yet generally maintains reliability, what obligations do those who develop and maintain that system have to us? If a particular product or service achieves such widespread adoption and reliability that it becomes integral to our cognitive functioning, could a sudden and significant change or a complete failure constitute a genuine cognitive impairment? The UN General Assembly's (non-binding) resolution in 2016, for example, recognizing that a government's intentional disruption of Internet access constitutes a form of coercion, underscores the fundamental role these technologies play in contemporary life and, arguably, within our extended minds.[5] Furthermore, we increasingly engage in the outsourcing of mental labor to automated systems, further blurring the lines between internal and external cognition.

Side quest: In the following scenarios, discuss who and/or what you believe is responsible for each of the following instances. Remember to be as *precise* as possible, and consider the objects or rather the products involved (hiPhone, ediPhone, etc.), and who or what is responsible for which parts of them:

- Your iPhone "bricks" (i.e., shuts down and cannot be turned back on). Presume you have some *very* important time-sensitive information there that you need access to right away (e.g., secret codes, a final paper, the greatest response in your group chat of all time);
- You have a document in a cloud-based note-taking service (e.g., iCloud Notes, Google Keep, MS OneNote, Evernote, Obsidian) on your phone and it's empty;
- You've been asked for some very important, time-sensitive information, and your texts aren't going through.

14.3.3 Where does the mind end and "AI" begin?

While the previous examples reflect our everyday realities and continue to raise complex philosophical questions, we're now encountering a more novel and potentially transformative class of technologies: generative and agentic systems. Although the full implications of these systems are still largely speculative, it is crucial that we consider their potential impact through the lens of EM.

Consider the role of an AI that assists in writing an essay (or maybe even this book!). Is this AI a sophisticated tool, or is it evolving into something more akin to a collaborator or a reliable partner in cognitive tasks? If so, do CL and AK need to add another co-author to this work?

When we rely on AI to provide answers to complex questions, where does our own intellectual contribution– our agency–begin and end? Are we exhibiting authorship, or does this reliance constitute a form of cognitive outsourcing that could border on plagiarism? Could these advanced AI systems eventually function as the "best tutor in the world," profoundly shaping our learning processes and modes of thinking? What becomes of our own agency and autonomy when we increasingly depend on these intelligent tools for decision-making and problem-solving?

Reflect on other technologies that have fundamentally reshaped our abilities and practices, such as digital cameras or automobiles. How might these more agentive systems compare in their transformative impact? Could we begin to conceptualize cognitive tasks in terms of "group work" where humans and AI systems collaboratively engage in intellectual endeavors? The empirical significance of EM emphasizes the impossibility of fully accounting for our thoughts without considering the surrounding apparatuses of enhancement, outsourcing, and abstraction. There's *plenty* to explore here. Here's just one example to get you going:

Side quest: Claude is our co-author?

Suppose a couple of philosophers (call them CL & AK) were writing a book. As they near the completion of their final chapters, they have a few ideas, arguments, and outlines sketched out, but get "stuck" trying to make their points flow and fit within the scope of the rest of the book.

Now let's say CL asks one of his colleagues, let's call him Claude, for a bit of help. He e-mails Claude their unfinished manuscript and says: "Hey Claude, we're looking for some feedback on how to flesh out these last couple of chapters. We've got the points and arguments we want to make sketched out, but we are stuck in developing them into a coherent narrative, keeping things within the scope of the book's primary aims, *and* doing so in the same tone of voice we've been writing in. We'd love any feedback or input you can offer! Thanks!"

Let's also say that AK does the exact same thing, but sends it to Claude™ the LLM. That is, AK gives Claude™ all the same context (docs, etc.) and makes the *exact* same request that CL does in his e-mail to Claude the colleague.

Claude the colleague, sees the e-mail, and decides he really wants to help CL and AK. He carefully reads the whole manuscript, and taking their specific considerations into account, takes a stab at fleshing out the unfinished chapters as best he can. He writes back to CL:

- "Hey Charlie! No problem. I looked at your attached work and took a stab at putting the unfinished drafts into something cohesive, based on what you'd specified. Here's what I came up with (see attached). Hope you like it!"

  Claude™, the LLM, receives the query, reviews the documents, takes their considerations into account, and gives AK a similar response:
- "Sure Aaron! No problem. I took a look at the documents and put the unfinished drafts into something cohesive, based on what you'd specified. Here's what I came up with (see attached). Hope you like it!"

So what's happened here? Who (or what) gets credit for authorship? Oftentimes, authors have an Acknowledgments section where they thank and give credit to folks for helping them with the book–reviewing early drafts, giving feedback, or helping out in any number of ways. Given the above situation, how should CL and AK handle the help they got from Claude and Claude™?

A natural place to start might be with: "it depends on how much of the output makes its way into the finished product." Either way, the authors have to decide, for instance, where acknowledgment ends and co-authorship begins. This gets tricky and may remind you of similar issues you've probably experienced doing *group work* or other collaborative projects. Placing "the right amounts of credit" where it's due can often be a nightmare (and believe us, it's a nightmare to grade too!). But now we're also talking about the outputs of humans versus AI systems (specifically large language models), and these "collaborators" certainly aren't human!

Who or what should receive acknowledgment or co-authorship in the following scenarios:

- We take the output "under consideration," are inspired by it (say, especially, the organization and structure), and keep it in mind as we write the unfinished chapters ourselves;
- We borrow specific sections of the output, copying and pasting a few sentences here and there, maybe even a whole paragraph or two, and massage the selected parts of the output a bit more to make them more in line with our objectives, thinking, and other things we might not have explicitly communicated yet;
- We're so satisfied with the output that we copy and paste it right over our existing unfinished chapters and call it a day;

Start by filling in the following chart, then articulate your reasons for your decision.

	Claude		*Claude™*	
	Acknowledgment	*Co-author*	*Acknowledgment*	*Co-author*
i.				
ii.				
iii.				

14.3.3.1 These examples viewed through a strongly embodied lens

How might the situations above look different when approached through a strong embodiment perspective? Recall from Section 6.2 our discussion of the causal–constitutive continuum and the parity principle from Chapter 4. These two ideas remind us that the line between "tools that merely *cause* thought" and "resources that literally *constitute* thought" is often blurry. Consider when someone makes an offhand comment that sparks a breakthrough idea. Did their remark simply cause you to think differently, or did it in some sense become part of the thought process itself, akin to Otto's reliance on his notebook? Emerging generative technologies such as large language models (LLMs) complicate this gray zone even further.

To bring this down to earth, think about group projects. Rarely do we declare with confidence that everyone contributed equally to a final paper or deliverable. Instead, authorship usually feels "vibes-based": some people clearly contributed more, others less, but exact contributions are difficult to measure. The same puzzle applies to technologies and tools. Even if we set aside agentic systems like LLMs, the question remains: how much credit (or authorship) belongs to the enabling tools and how much belongs to us humans?

Typically, we don't thank or acknowledge the mundane infrastructure that made our work possible. CL and AK don't credit our Internet service provider, the Google Docs platform, or Zoom for helping us collaborate on this very book. Cormac McCarthy never thanked his typewriter for helping him write his books, even though it was the immediate material condition of his novels; it would be weird if he did. His now-famous Olivetti Lettera 32 typewriter sold for over $25,000 at auction. Was there something special or magical about this product such that it enabled him to write incredible literature and win the Nobel Prize? Probably not; he later went out and bought another typewriter for $11 and managed to write more award-winning literature.[6] It's more likely that his typewriter's mystique came not from intrinsic magical properties but from its coupling with McCarthy's *expertise*.

What matters, then, is not the sheer presence of a tool, but how it meshes with cognitive systems. This was a point raised in Section 6.2: the details of interaction, relation, and patterned expertise determine whether something sits on the merely causal side of the spectrum or crosses into the constitutive. The parity principle challenges us to ask: if an external process plays the same reliable role as an internal one, why not treat it as genuinely cognitive?

In this sense, authorship, cognition, and technological mediation all require attention to the fine-grained texture of use. Minds and technologies do not meet at a single clear boundary; rather, they are stitched together through ongoing couplings. Whether in collaborative writing, group projects, or the integration of AI tools, what ultimately matters is how these systems interlock to extend our capacities. That is the strong embodiment perspective: cognition is not simply housed inside the head but enacted across tools, people, and environments in ways that challenge easy causal explanations.

14.3.4 Haptics

Recall our earlier discussions concerning the body in action and the active nature of perception. One of the most effective ways to learn and gain understanding is through direct engagement and physical interaction. Examining haptics—the sense of touch—through the framework of EM presents intriguing possibilities for understanding how technology can become more deeply integrated with our embodied cognition.

Consider how the use of a tool can extend our sense of bodily awareness. Maurice Merleau-Ponty, in his seminal work *Phenomenology of Perception*, provided the well-known example of the blind man's cane. This concept can be readily grasped by simply picking up a pen or pencil and using it to "feel around" your environment. You will likely notice how the pen begins to feel like an extension of your hand, enabling you to perceive and interact with objects in a novel way. The pen doesn't have a mind, nor does it have any neurons or sensory receptors that run through it. But the fascinating bit here is that through reliable coupling and active exploration, the perceived boundaries of your own body seem to expand to encompass the tool. This aligns with the EM perspective that manipulating the physical world directly influences our cognitive and mental landscape.

Now think about this in terms of the development of haptic technology. The above aspect of perception (known in part as "extension" in phenomenology) is leveraged to create the experience of engaging with things that aren't directly in front of us, like feeling an object in VR or remotely coming into contact with objects far away from us. Roughly speaking, we use tactile sensations like vibration, motion, or force to create a sense of touch, enhancing one's experience and interactions with devices, virtual environments, and even remote control of machinery. This technology has been around for some time, but it's *very* expensive (especially the hardware bit) and thus typically used in specialized scenarios.

The "analog" version of this is as old as teaching itself. Think of how you might have learned to hit a baseball, ride a bicycle, or swing a golf club. It's likely someone put their arms around you and moved or "puppeted" your body so that you accomplished the task better. You got a feel for things like timing, body position, and coordinated motions—all things that fall into the category of *implicit* (non-propositional) knowledge, that is, know-how, as we first saw in Section 6.3.3. To gain know-how, this has been one of the best methods to date.

Side quest: Take any task that requires a lot of know-how, like driving a stick shift, hitting a golf ball, or riding a motorcycle. If you know how to do any of these things, try teaching it to someone who doesn't, using only propositional knowledge—i.e., by explaining it in sentences or through written descriptions. Suppose you explain it as clearly and completely as possible, and your student is also the *best* student, and remembers everything you said. Do you think they'll be able to accomplish the task now? Would you, for example, give them the keys to your car or motorcycle and let them take it for a spin?

Suppose there was a different way to teach people things like this, one where we used haptics. An instructor or professional might remotely control us to move in the right sorts of ways at the right times. Rather than someone yelling instructions from a distance, like "keep your elbows up" and "OK. Swing now!", no words would need to be exchanged, but you'd be learning a *lot*. This could help scaffold the acquisition of know-how. If there were, say, a "haptic wetsuit" that let a pro surfer move me while I was in the water, maybe, just maybe, my timing and form would improve and I'd become a better surfer.

14.4 Wrapping up: ethical considerations and the future

As technology becomes increasingly interwoven with our cognitive lives, we must grapple with the profound ethical implications that arise. The fundamental principle that manipulating the physical world also influences the cognitive and mental realm takes on new significance in this context.

The outsourcing of mental labor to technological systems can undoubtedly free up valuable cognitive resources, potentially allowing us to focus on other tasks or pursue new intellectual endeavors. However, we must also carefully consider the potential long-term effects of this reliance on our own cognitive abilities. If our extended cognitive systems were to become unreliable due to technical failures or be altered without our informed consent, what would be the consequences for our autonomy, sense of self, and our overall well-being? Our analogy drawn earlier between service interruptions and neural ablations underscores the potential for significant impact. The issues from chapters 12 and 13 take on a new life in this context.

Furthermore, as we continue to develop more agentive technologies, fundamental questions concerning responsibility, authorship, and control become paramount. We need to establish clear ethical guidelines and carefully consider the distinction between a helpful tool and a system that could ultimately undermine our own agency, critical thinking skills, and understanding of the world around us.

14.5 Conclusion

While Socrates's concerns about the advent of writing may appear somewhat antiquated in our technologically saturated world, they highlight a persistent and deeply human concern about how novel technologies shape our minds and ways of knowing. By carefully applying the lens of extended mind to specific products and services, we can move beyond simplistic and often polarized perspectives on technology toward a more nuanced understanding of its profound impact. Our technological devices, when reliably coupled with us and integrated into our daily practices, can indeed function as integral components of our extended minds. However, this cognitive extension is not without ramifications, ranging from the definition of our cognitive processes to the ethical responsibilities of those who design, develop, and maintain these increasingly vital systems. As technology continues its rapid and often unpredictable evolution, the frameworks of embodied and extended cognition provide us with conceptual tools for navigating this complex relationship between human beings and the technologies that are increasingly shaping our lives.

Notes

1 Yes, in those times, the entirety of Homer's Odyssey, for example, was committed to memory. But certainly not today (at least we don't know anyone who has memorized the whole thing).
2 Chatfield, Tom. 2024. *Wise Animals: How Technology Has Made Us What We Are*. Picador. (p. 71).
3 In Chalmers' foreward to Clark's (2008) book *Supersizing the Mind*, he says flat out that "[t]he iPhone is part of my mind already"–(Clark 2008, p. ix).
4 It's absurd to talk about things like patch updates, feature rollouts, or service issues for an old-fashioned paper notebook (like Otto's), or that one's notebook "dies" because it runs out of battery.
5 Cf. Article 19 resolution and the topic of the Right to Internet Access
6 https://www.wired.com/2009/12/cormac-mccarthys-typewriter-dies-after-50-years-and-five-million-words/

15

FUTURE DIRECTIONS

Embodied cognition has a long and storied history. We've discussed only the last few decades. Some philosophers have suggested that we can find implicit or explicit statements about embodiment in the Western tradition in Aristotle, St. Thomas Aquinas, and Spinoza. In the twentieth century, philosophers like Husserl, Merleau-Ponty, Sartre, and Heidegger emphasized the central role of the body in perception, action, and thought.

All of that is to say: in focusing primarily on work done since the late twentieth century, we've only scratched the surface of what there is to think about the embodied mind. There is so much more to read, explore, and debate.

Throughout this book, we've tried to show that embodied cognition has implications that extend beyond how we understand the relationship between mind and body. We've considered its significance for free will, ethics, and technology. In this final chapter, we turn to two more areas of active and promising research: mental health and culture.

15.1 Mental health and embodiment[1]

We've alluded several times to hanger: being angry as a result of being hungry. This is an easy go-to example of the impact of the body on your mental wellbeing. Other examples here are easy to find: drinking water, getting sufficient sleep, exercise, and eating fruits and veggies are also ways that you can take care of your body that have an impact on your mental health.

But there are other, and more subtle ways of looking at the role of the body in mental health. One well-regarded book on the subject is Bessel van

DOI: 10.4324/9781003356622-18

der Kolk's *The Body Keeps the Score*. In it, van der Kolk describes the effects that trauma has on the body, particularly the brain. He laments what he calls the "pharmacological revolution" as a myopic way of coping with trauma. On the whole, van der Kolk has done a lot to highlight the importance of embodiment for mental health. We aren't brains in meat suits. We are embodied organisms located in an environment.

Nonetheless, as a philosophical point, we're skeptical of the ways in which van der Kolk describes his findings. He seems to fall into the sort of brain-body dualism we mentioned in Section 4.2. He describes on pp. 206–207, for instance, the "rational brain, which expresses itself in thoughts." But by the same token, he talks about "gut feelings" and behaviors. Though we may be a little grumpy with the metaphysics, this is a case where the metaphysics and the sciences can be mutually informative.

In talking about traumatic memories, van der Kolk notes that they are different from other kinds of memories. You might remember what you had for breakfast or what you did on your sixth birthday. Traumatic memories "inhabit" the body in a way different from other sorts of memories. For example, people who suffer from post-traumatic stress disorder (PTSD) experience triggering feelings in a way different from other sorts of memories. Such people have a hard time distinguishing past threats from present situations. When the veteran hears or sees something that triggers memories of their experiences of war, the body responds in ways very similar to how it would respond if they were actually at war. The bodily responses to triggering stimuli are much more intense; for the person having those responses, the experience of the world differs dramatically. Van der Kolk notes that one way to begin recovering from such traumatic memories is to reclaim a sense of ownership of one's body through mindfulness practices like yoga. The person afflicted with PTSD comes to "inhabit" their body in a new way; their experience of their body changes.

Aside from van der Kolk's work in clinical psychology, we find philosophers developing new concepts for mental health and illness. Consider, for instance, autism spectrum disorder (ASD), which is characterized by difficulty in social interaction and communication. One well-discussed explanation for ASD appeals to an internal process called **mindreading**: inferring the mental states of another person given your observations of their behaviors (first seen in Section 10.5). Someone with ASD is not able to mindread in the same way as most neurotypical folks. Krueger (2021) proposes instead that ASD is characterized by *style-blindness*. When we perceive people's behaviors, we have an intuitive and implicit grasp on the manner, or *style*, of an action: you can tell when someone is sad, for example, by picking up on their bodily posture and movement. You might even say that we have something like expert-level knowledge of styles of action (see Section 12.9).

Folks with ASD have a difficult time picking up on the style of actions performed by neurotypical agents. That's to say: they are style-blind.

Here is one more example of philosophers developing concepts of embodiment for use in clinical psychology. Erik Rietveld and Julian Kiverstein (2014) make an interesting suggestion toward the end of their paper, "A Rich Landscape of Affordances." They allude to an interpretation of depressive experiences in which the affordances perceived become flattened and grey. Nothing stands out as meaningful or valuable. There is little in the way of emotional responses or sense-making in the perception of the world. Maiese (2020) describes the characteristic symptom of depression in terms of affect and time. She suggests that our typical engagements with the world are emotion-laden and future-directed: we go about our lives sensitive to emotions evoked and thinking toward the future.[2] This sense of future-directedness for individuals experiencing depression is disrupted: there's no sense of meaningfulness in the future.

These different takes on mental health and illness are important because they suggest different ways to heal. Maiese, for example, suggests dance and art as two ways of reclaiming the sense that there is meaningfulness in the future. Through the arts, one's sense of meaningfulness in the future can be restored. This strongly contrasts with the psychopharmacological approach.[3]

15.1.1 Mental health and metatheory

We mentioned that we are a little grumpy that van der Kolk doesn't stay in one theoretical lane. His conceptual framework slides between weak and strong embodiment and may even dip its toes into disembodiment! Still, we think his work in this context provides a helpful lesson for thinking about the embodied mind in applied settings.

There are times when practice doesn't always match up with theory. Remember Immanuel Kant from Section 13.4? He argued that no one may ever lie, even to save a life.[4] This is a case where the theory doesn't quite match our intuitions about what we should do. So what do we do? Do we give up the theory or do we change our intuitions about when it's okay to lie?

In a similar vein, van der Kolk talks about the mind, in at least some cases, in a disembodied way. So what do we do? Do we cast a suspicious eye on this area of van der Kolk's work because he doesn't respect theoretical boundaries?[5] Or do we ignore the theoretical boundaries if van der Kolk's approach actually works? In other words, if it turns out some conceptualizations of mental health mean acting *as if* the mind is disembodied, do we adjust our theory to fit the practice or do we adjust our practice to fit the theory? Or do we do neither and let the chips fall where they may?

These are hard questions and no answer is obvious. Each answer has advantages and drawbacks. The only thing that's clear is that wrestling with these questions is unavoidable and difficult.

Now you might recall the Spectrum view in Section 11.1: no token case of cognition is either entirely extended or entirely unextended, but always falls somewhere in between. This is a metatheoretical possibility that van der Kolk can adopt. If treating cases like they're mostly disembodied works best, then do that. But if treating cases like mostly strongly embodied works best, then do that instead. The theory of embodiment that's adopted is determined by which has the greatest practical benefit at the time.[6] The trouble is that there's a real human cost to this kind of theoretical looseness; but then again, those costs may be unavoidable given the relatively new fields of abnormal psychology and psychiatric treatment for mental illness.

15.2 Culture and embodiment

Another place we see embodied cognition developing is with respect to culture. We've covered a little of this already. Conceptual metaphor theory (CMT), introduced in Section 7.4.2.1, is one way to incorporate culture into embodiment. Remember that the foundational idea of CMT is that we think in metaphors, like HAPPY IS UP and ARGUMENT IS WAR. Some of these metaphors are informed by culture. Consider one of its examples: TIME IS MONEY. Money is certainly a cultural concept; there's no money without some kind of culture! Our concepts—the building blocks of thought—are informed by culture as well as our embodied experience.

But that's not all! There are lines of research suggesting that cultures are responses to environmental pressures. In other words, cultures are the way they are—at least in part—because of the environment. Two major cultural features are **individualism** and **collectivism**, mentioned in a Sidequest in Section 12.8. People in individualist cultures—like those of America, Canada, and New Zealand, among others—tend to put the good of the individual ahead of the good of the group. Boundaries between in-groups and out-groups are loose and flexible, and the sense of self excludes others. They're prone to analytic thinking—decomposing problems in order to solve them a piece at a time. They tend to be emotionally expressive, at least compared to folks from collectivist cultures. Collectivist cultures—found in China, Japan, and South Korea, among others—tend to put the good of the group ahead of the good of the individual. There are firm in-group and out-group boundaries, and the sense of self includes others. They incline toward holistic thinking—considering lots of information as a whole, even when some of that information is contradictory. They also tend to be emotionally reserved.[7]

So what sorts of environmental conditions would provoke individualist or collectivist cultures? Let's consider collectivist cultures first. Growing rice requires *a lot* of collaboration among neighbors. Farmers have to make collective decisions about major issues like when to flood the rice paddies. This means that rice farmers have to be pretty tolerant of their neighbors, putting up with them when they are annoying and sometimes withholding expressions of frustration. This is for the good of the group: if you can't put aside your annoyances with your neighbor and work with them, then you and others might go hungry. Researchers find that East Asian cultures, where rice is a dietary staple, tend to do exactly this: reserve expressions of emotion and put the good of the whole ahead of the individual's good. Where rice is a dietary staple, adopting collectivist tendencies is crucial for survival.

Compare this with cultures of growing wheat. It's hard work and there's a lot to be done, but it doesn't require the same kind of coordination that farming rice does. You don't need to work with other wheat farmers to time your harvest. You just go and harvest. If you're a wheat farmer, you don't need to be as reserved in your emotional expressions because you don't have to work as closely with other people. If you're annoyed with your neighbor, you can be mad about it all day long. They're not around (usually), so let your anger out! Researchers find that Western cultures where wheat is a staple tend to be more emotionally expressive.[8] That's to say, folks from individualist cultures can prioritize their own well-being and let it all out.

One more example. Cultures in high-pathogen areas tend to be collectivist, maintaining robust in-group and out-group boundaries. Why? Suppose you live in a place where there are all kinds of nasty viruses and bacteria floating around, waiting to take you down. The safe strategy in this kind of environment is to stick with the people you know aren't sick and to be wary of anyone from outside your community. After all, if some stranger comes into your community, who knows what kinds of pathogens they might be carrying? Keeping the group safe means being hostile (or at least very unfriendly) to outsiders.[9]

Now, given all of that, how do we fit culture into the mechanisms of embodiment? One way is to follow Alvin Goldman and accept weak embodiment. Here, you fit culture into mental representations and mental processes. Figuring out how all this works in the brain will be hard, but the conceptual questions are more or less clear. We saw some of this work in Chapter 7.

But suppose you find strong embodiment more compelling. What then? One way you can go (but certainly not the only way) is to develop cultural "versions" of concepts introduced in Chapter 9. For example, consider the idea of *cultural affordances*. We've seen something like this already with *social* affordances, but social features and cultural features don't overlap entirely: New Yorkers and Texans are both Americans even though they don't share the same social norms and expectations. What cultural affordances might they both pick up on? We can look to **cultural psychology** for help in answering this question. Americans are highly individualistic, putting personal goals ahead of group goals. So cultural affordances for Americans are affordances that resonate with individualistic ideals. Moving a thousand miles away from your parents is something doable for many Americans. If it's not practically doable, it's at least conceivable. Compare this with collectivist cultures, like Taiwan or Japan, where moving thousands of miles from home is less of a genuine possibility. The term for this is *residential mobility*. People from individualistic cultures have a higher sense of residential mobility than people from collectivist cultures.[10] That is, the affordances for relocation vary with culture.

The concept of a cultural affordance also connects with expectations we have of others. In addition to residential mobility there is *relational mobility*: how free people feel to begin and end relationships. In the USA (and many Western nations), there are high degrees of relational mobility. You make new friends and lose touch with old ones. That's just how things go. Relationships are based on shared interests and mutual attraction (emotional, social, physical, etc.). You might be sad when one of your close childhood friends starts running with a different crowd and you have a falling-out, but it's a fairly normal occurrence. By contrast, East Asian cultures have lower degrees of relational mobility. The likelihood of ending relationships, especially long-standing ones, is much lower. A colleague of mine (CL) raised in Japan once mentioned that he and his childhood best friend have nothing in common, but they're best friends nonetheless. Again, we might think about relational mobility in terms of cultural affordances. Some cultures afford moving in and out of relationships more easily than others.

Even setting aside creating cultural "versions" of some strong embodiment concepts, cultural patterns point to interesting questions. Connected to relational mobility, expectations for how we interact with others vary with culture.[11] In high relational mobility cultures, people have to work harder to get and keep friends. A person can display their value as a partner by being generous. A person can also signal trust in another by divulging personal information. In romantic relationships, passionate love is more important in high relational mobility cultures: it signals valuing of and commitment to your partner. Basically, in high relational mobility cultures, your partner (romantic or platonic) is free to leave, so you have to work to keep them around. Expectations people have of others will vary across cultures. What does this mean for participatory sense-making? What does it mean for emotional expression and empathy?

15.3 Conclusion

This is all just a teaser. There is so much more to think about with respect to embodiment and its applications. As we learn more about the mind, body, and environment, we'll return again and again to old problems with fresh insights. And as our technology develops, we'll reflect more and more about our embodiment and just what it is that makes us human. We close with the immortal words of C.M. Burns:

> In closing, gentle reader, I'd like to thank you. What's that you say? Me thanking you? No, it's not a misprint. For you see, I enjoyed writing this book as much as you enjoyed reading it.[12]

Notes

1 Many thanks to Hailey O'Hara for her assistance in collecting the materials and talking through the content of this section.

2 For example, your love for your friend helps you make sense of the world and orient yourself toward the future—namely, a future in which you can do things motivated by your love for your friend.

3 Of course, if you find yourself experiencing these sorts of feelings, you should put down this book and talk with someone, preferably a mental health professional.

4 "On a Supposed Right to Lie from Benevolent Concerns" is the essay in question. Many Kant scholars either (i) ignore this essay, casting it as a misstep by Kant, or (ii) argue that the allegedly absurd conclusion is a misinterpretation. For discussion of Kant on this point, see the essays, "Kant and Overdemandingness I: The Demandingness of Imperfect Duties" (Saunders, Slater, and Sticker 2024) and "Kant and Overdemandingness II: The Demandingness of Perfect Duties" (Saunders, Slater, and Sticker 2025).

5 Another way of putting this is to ask: Should van der Kolk rethink his analyses where he drifts into disembodiment?

6 This view has connections with **American pragmatism**, a philosophical position that asks about the practical value of a belief or claim. The relevance of practical value varies from one pragmatist to another, but it's never entirely absent.

7 There are simplifications here of complex and nuanced cultures. Even within cultures, there's a lot of variation. If you're an American, you can imagine differences between New Yorkers and residents of Wilbur, WA. It's a town of roughly 900 people (as of 2024) in Eastern Washington, 65 miles from Spokane (population roughly 231,000) and 230 miles from Seattle (population roughly 781,000). Even with the variations within cultures, the data suggest that the patterns we discuss in this section tend to hold for members of the respective cultures.

8 Talhelm, T. (2020). "Emerging Evidence of Cultural Differences Linked to Rice Versus Wheat Agriculture," *Current Opinion in Psychology* 32, 87–88. Talhelm notes that people in collectivist cultures aren't necessarily nicer or friendlier (i.e., "prosocial"). They have tighter connections among community members, which comes with greater obligations.

9 Vukov and Lassiter (2020) use this case as a way to motivate a culture-friendly metaphysics of mind.

10 Oishi, S. ad Choi, H. (2020). "The Psychology of Residential Mobility: A Decade of Progress," *Current Opinion in Psychology* 32, 72–75.

11 Yuki, M. & Schug, J. (2020). "Psychological Consequences of Relational Mobility," *Current Opinion in Psychology* 32: 129–132.

12 From *Will There Ever Be a Rainbow*, in *The Simpsons*, "Blood Feud," season 2, episode 22.

WORKS CITED

Abraham, Ralph and Christopher Shaw. *Dynamics: The Geometry of Behavior*, 5th ed. Aerial Press, 2016.

Adams, Fred and Ken Aizawa. *The Bounds of Cognition*. Blackwell, 2008.

Adams, Fred and Ken Aizawa. "Defending the bounds of cognition." In *The Extended Mind*, edited by Richard Menary. The MIT Press, 2010, 67–80.

Alsmith, Adrian John Tetteh, and Frédérique De Vignemont. "Embodying the mind and representing the body." *Review of Philosophy and Psychology* 3, no. 1 (2012): 1–13.

Anderson, M. L.. *After Phrenology: Neural Reuse and the Interactive Brain*. MIT Press, 2014a.

Anderson, S. L. (Ed.). *The Cambridge Handbook of Artificial Intelligence*. Cambridge University Press, 2014b.

Arango, Alejandro, and Adam Burgos. "The social identity affordance view: A theory of social identities." *The Southern Journal of Philosophy* 62, no. 2 (2024): 162–177.

Baggs, Edward. "All affordances are social: Foundations of a Gibsonian social ontology." *Ecological Psychology* 33, no. 3–4 (2021): 257–278.

Bering, Jesse M. "The folk psychology of souls." *Behavioral and Brain Sciences* 29, no. 5 (2006): 453–462. https://doi.org/10.1017/S0140525X06009101

Bruner, Jerome. *Acts of Meaning*. Harvard University Press, 1990.

Chalmers, D. J. The singularity: A philosophical analysis. *Journal of Consciousness Studies* 17 (2010): 7–65.

Chatfield, Tom. *Wise Animals: How Technology Has Made Us What We Are*. Picador, 2024.

Chemero, Anthony. *Radical Embodied Cognitive Science*. The MIT Press, 2009.

Chomsky, Noam "Review of *Verbal behavior* by B.F. Skinner." *Language* 1 (1959): 26–58.

Clark, A. *Being there: Putting Brain, Body, and World Together Again*. MIT Press, 1997.

Clark, A. *Natural-born Cyborgs: Minds, Technologies, and the Future of Human Intelligence*. Oxford University Press, 2003.

Clark, A. *Supersizing the Mind: Embodiment, Action, and Cognitive Extension.* Oxford University Press, 2008.
Clark, A. "Coupling, constitution, and the cognitive kind: A reply to Adams and Aizawa." In *The Extended Mind*, edited by R. Menary. The MIT Press, 2010, 81–100.
Clark, A., and Chalmers, D. J. "The extended mind." *Analysis* 58, no. 1 (1998): 7–19.
de Bruin, L., Strijbos, D., and Slors, M. "Situating emotions: From embodied cognition to mindreading." *Topoi* 34 (2015): 469–479.
De Jaegher, Hanne, and Ezequiel Di Paolo. "Participatory sense-making: An enactive approach to social cognition." *Phenomenology and the Cognitive Sciences* 6, no. 4 (2007): 485–507.
DeSousa, Ronald. *The Rationality of Emotion*. The MIT Press, 1987.
Deacon, T. W. *The Symbolic Species: The Co-evolution of Language and the Brain.* W.W. Norton & Company, 1997.
Dennett, Daniel. "The nature of images and the introspective trap." In *Content and Consciousness*. Routledge, 1968, 132–140.
Drayson, Z. "What is action-oriented perception?" In *Logic, Methodology and Philosophy of Science: Proceedings of the 15th International Congress*, edited by D. Zoe. College Publications, 2017. https://philarchive.org/rec/DRAWIA-3
Fodor, Jerry. "Where is my mind?" *London Review of Books* 31, no.3 (2009): 13–15.
Fodor, Jerry. *Modularity of Mind*. The MIT Press, 1983.
Frankfurt, H. G. "Freedom of the will and the concept of a person." *Journal of Philosophy* 68, no. 1 (1971): 5–20.
Gallagher, Shaun. *How the Body Shapes the Mind*. Oxford University Press, 2005.
Gallagher, Shaun. *Enactivist Interventions*. Oxford University Press, 2017.
Gibson, J. J. *The Senses Considered as Perceptual Systems*. Houghton Mifflin, 1966.
Gibson, J. J. *The Ecological Approach to Visual Perception*. Houghton Mifflin, 1979.
Glenberg, Arthur M., and Michael P. Kaschak. "Grounding language in action." *Psychonomic Bulletin & Review* 9, no. 3 (2002): 558–565.
Goldman, A. I. "A moderate approach to embodied cognitive science." *Review of Philosophy and Psychology* 2, no. 3 (2011): 555–569.
Goldman, A. "The bodily formats approach to embodied cognition." In *Current Controversies in the Philosophy of Mind*, edited by U. Kriegel. Routledge, 2014.
Goldman, Alvin, and Frédérique De Vignemont. "Is social cognition embodied?." *Trends in Cognitive Sciences* 13, no. 4 (2009): 154–159.
Greenemeier, L. "20 years after deep blue: how AI has advanced since conquering chess." 2017. http://www.scientificamerican.com/article/20-years-after-deep-blue-how-ai-has-advanced-since-conquering-chess/. Accessed 29 September 2025.
Heersmink, R. "The internet, cognitive enhancement, and the values of cognition." *Minds and Machines* 26, no. 4 (2016): 389–407.
Heft, H. *Ecological Psychology in Context: James Gibson, Roger Barker, and the Legacy of William James's Radical Empiricism*. Lawrence Erlbaum Associates, 2001.
Heine, S. J., Lehman, D. R., Markus, H. R., and Kitayama, S. "Is there a universal need for positive self-regard?" *Psychological Review* 106, no. 4 (1999): 766–794.
Hutto, D. D., and Myin, E. *Radicalizing Enactivism: Basic Minds without Content.* MIT Press, 2012.
Hutto, D. D., and Myin, E. *Evolving Enactivism*. MIT Press, 2017.

Jackson, Frank. "What Mary Didn't Know." *The Journal of Philosophy* 83, no. 5 (1986): 291. https://doi.org/10.2307/2026143
Japyassú, Hilton F., and Kevin Laland. "Extended spider cognition." *Animal Cognition* 20 (2017): 375–395.
James, William. *The Principles of Psychology*, vol 1 and 2. Dover Publications, Inc., 1950. (Originally published in 1890).
Jaworski, William. *Philosophy of Mind: A Comprehensive Introduction.* Wiley-Blackwell, 2011.
Johnson, M. *Moral Imagination: Implications of Cognitive Science for Ethics.* University of Chicago Press, 1993.
Kane, R. *A Contemporary Introduction to Free Will.* Oxford University Press, 2005.
Krueger, Joel. "Enactivism, Other Minds, and Mental Disorders." *Synthese* 198, no. Suppl 1 (2021): 365–389.
Lakoff, G., and Johnson, M. *Metaphors We Live By.* University of Chicago Press, 1980.
Legg, Catherine, and Jack Reynolds. "Habits of mind. New insights for embodied cognition from classical pragmatism and phenomenology." *European Journal of Pragmatism and American Philosophy* 14, no. XIV-2 (2022). https://journals.openedition.org/ejpap/2994
Maiese, M. *Embodiment, Emotion, and Cognition.* Palgrave Macmillan, 2011.
Maiese, Michelle. "An enactivist approach to treating depression: Cultivating online intelligence through dance and music." *Phenomenology and the Cognitive Sciences* 19, no. 3 (2020): 523–547.
Mandik, Pete. "Action-oriented representation." In *Cognition and the Brain: The Philosophy and Neuroscience Movement*, edited by Andrew Brook and Kathleen Akins, 2005, 284–305.
Markus, H. and Kitayama, S. "Culture and the self: Implications for cognition, emotion, and motivation." *Psychological Review* 98, no. 2 (1991): 224–253.
Marr, D. *Vision: A Computational Investigation into the Human Representation and Processing of Visual Information.* W.H. Freeman, 1982.
Maxwell, Nicholas. "Physics and common sense." *The British Journal for the Philosophy of Science* 16, no. 64 (1966): 295–311.
McCulloch, Warren S., and Walter Pitts. "A logical calculus of the ideas immanent in nervous activity." *The Bulletin of Mathematical Biophysics* 5, no. 4 (1943): 115–133.
Merleau-Ponty, M. *Phenomenology of Perception.* Trans. D. A. Landes. Routledge, 2012. (Original work published 1945).
Miller, George. "The magical number seven, plus or minus two: Some limits on our capacity for processing information." *Psychological Review* 63(1956): 81–97.
Morrison, J. *Cleanse Your Body, Clear your Mind.* G.P. Putnam's Sons, 2010.
Nanay, Bence. "Entity realism about mental representations." *Erkenntnis* 87, no. 1 (2022): 75–91.
Nichols, M. James, and William T. Newsome. "The neurobiology of cognition." *Nature* 402, no. Suppl 6761 (1999): C35–C38.
Nisbett, R. *The Geography of Thought.* Free Press, 2003.
Noë, A. *Action in Perception.* MIT Press, 2004.
Noë, A. "The enactive approach: a briefer statement, with some remarks on "radical enactivism"." *Phenomenology and the Cognitive Sciences* 20 (2021): 957–970.
O'Regan, J. K. *Why Red Doesn't Sound like a Bell: Understanding the Feel of Consciousness.* Oxford University Press, 2011.

O'Regan, J. K., and Noë, A. "A sensorimotor account of vision and visual consciousness." *Behavioral and Brain Sciences* 24, no. 5 (2001): 939–973.
Pereboom, Derk. "Free will skepticism and criminal punishment." In *The Future of Punishment*, edited by Thomas Nadelhoffer. Oxford University Press, 2013, 49–78.
Proudfoot, Diane. "Rethinking Turing's test." *The Journal of Philosophy* 110, no. 7 (2013): 391–411.
Putnam, Hilary. "The mental life of some machines." In *Mind, Language, and Reality: Philosophical Papers, volume 2*. Cambridge University Press, 1975, 408–428.
Prinz, J. *Furnishing the Mind: Concepts and their Perceptual Basis*. MIT Press, 2002.
Prinz, J. *Gut Reactions: A Perceptual Theory of Emotion*. Oxford University Press, 2004.
Prinz, J. *The Emotional Construction of Morals*. Oxford University Press, 2007.
Pulvermüller, Friedemann. "Brain mechanisms linking language and action." *Nature Reviews Neuroscience* 6, no. 7 (2005): 576–582.
Rietveld, Erik, and Julian Kiverstein. "A rich landscape of affordances." *Ecological Psychology* 26, no. 4 (2014): 325–352.
Shweder, Richard (Ed.) *Welcome to Middle Age! (And Other Cultural Fictions)*. Chicago University Press, 1998.
Ryle, Gilbert. *The Concept of Mind*. Barnes & Noble Books, 1949.
Saunders, J., Slater, J., and Sticker, M. (2024), "Kant and overdemandingness I: The demandingness of imperfect duties." *Philosophy Compass*, e12998. https://doi.org/10.1111/phc3.12998
Saunders, J., Slater, J. and Sticker, M. (2025), "Kant and overdemandingness II: The demandingness of perfect duties." *Philosophy Compass* 20: e70033. https://doi.org/10.1111/phc3.70033
Solomon, R. C. *The Passions: Emotions and the Meaning of Life*. Hackett Publishing Company, 1993.
Sokolowski, R. *Introduction to Phenomenology*. Cambridge University Press, 2000.
Strawson, G. "The impossibility of moral responsibility." *Philosophical Studies* 75, nos. 1–2 (1994): 5–24.
Strawson, P. F.. "Self, mind and body." In *Freedom and Resentment and Other Essays*. Routledge, 2008, 186–195. (Originally published in 1974.)
Stich, Stephen and Ted Warfield, eds. *Mental Representation: A Reader*. Basil Blackwell, 1994.
Sutton, John. "Exograms and interdisciplinarity." In *The Extended Mind*, edited by R. Menary. The MIT Press, 2010, 189–225.
Talhelm, T. "Emerging evidence of cultural differences linked to rice versus wheat agriculture." *Current Opinion in Psychology* 32 (2020): 87–88
Thompson, E. *Mind in Life: Biology, Phenomenology, and the Sciences of Mind*. Belknap Press of Harvard University Press, 2007.
Trnka, Radek, and Radmila Lorencova. "Indigenous concepts of consciousness, soul, and spirit: A cross-cultural perspective." *Journal of Consciousness Studies* 29, no. 1–2 (2022): 113–140.
Turing, Alan Mathison. "On computable numbers, with an application to the *Entscheidungsproblem*." *Journal of Mathematics* 58 (1936): 345–363.
Turing, Alan M. "Computing machinery and intelligence (1950)." *Mind* 59, no. 236 (1950): 433–460.

van Inwagen, P. "The incompatibility of free will and determinism." *Philosophical Studies* 27, no. 3 (1975): 185–199.

Varela, Francisco, Evan Thompson, and Eleanor Rosch. *The Embodied Mind: Cognitive Science and Human Experience*, revised ed. The MIT Press, 1991.

von Uexküll, J. *A Foray into the Worlds of Animals and Humans*. Trans. J. D. O'Neil. University of Minnesota Press, 2010.

Vukov, Joseph, and Charles Lassiter. "How to power encultured minds." *Synthese* 197, no. 8 (2020): 3507–3534.

Wilson, Andrew D., and Sabrina Golonka. "Embodied cognition is not what you think it is." *Frontiers in Psychology* 4 (2013), article 58.

Wittgenstein, Ludwig. *Tractatus Logico-Philosophicus*, 2nd ed. Trans. D. F. Pears and B. F. McGuinness. Routledge, 2001a. (Originally published in 1922.)

Wittgenstein, Ludwig. *Philosophical Investigations*. Translated by G.E.M. Anscombe. Blackwell Publishers, 2001b.

Wittgenstein, Ludwig. *Philosophical Investigations*, revised 4th ed. Ed. P. M. S. Hacker and Joachim Schulte. Trans. G. E. M. Anscombe, P. M. S. Hacker and Joachim Schulte. Blackwell Publishing, 2009. (Originally published in 1953.)

Zahavi, D. *Phenomenology: The Basics*. Routledge, 2019.

SUGGESTED READING

Chapter 1: Introduction

Blackburn, Simon. *Think: A Compelling Introduction to Philosophy*. New York: Oxford University Press, 2013.

de Cruz, Helen. *Philosophy Illustrated*. New York: Oxford University Press, 2021.

Russell, Bertrand. *The Problems of Philosophy*. London: Oxford University Press, 1959.

Sousanis, Nick. *Unflattening*. Cambridge, MA: Harvard University Press, 2015.

Chapter 2: From Aporia to Philosophy

Churchland, Paul M. *Matter and Consciousness*. Revised ed. Cambridge, MA: The MIT Press, 1988.

Descartes, René. *Discourse on Method and Meditations on First Philosophy*. Translated by Donald A. Cress. 4th ed. Indianapolis, IN: Hackett Publishing Company, 1998.

Gertler, Brie. "In defense of mind-body dualism." *Journal of Philosophy* 79, no. 8 (1982): 419–439.

Kim, Jaegwon. *Philosophy of Mind*. 3rd ed. Boulder, CO: Westview Press, 2011.

Levin, Janet, "Functionalism." In *The Stanford Encyclopedia of Philosophy* (Summer 2023 Edition). Edited by Edward N. Zalta and Uri Nodelman. https://plato.stanford.edu/archives/sum2023/entries/functionalism/

McWeeny, Jen. "Princess Elisabeth and the mind-body problem." In *Just the Arguments: 100 of the Most Important Arguments in Western Philosophy*. Edited by Michael Bruce and Steven Barbone. New York: Wiley-Blackwell, 2011, 297–300.

Weiskopf, Daniel and Fred Adams. *An Introduction to the Philosophy of Psychology*. New York: Cambridge University Press, 2015.

Chapter 3: Rise and Fall of Disembodiment

Boden, Margaret. *Mind as Machine: A History of Cognitive Science*. 2 vols. Oxford; New York: Oxford University Press, 2006.

Churchland, Patricia S. *Neurophilosophy: Toward a Unified Science of the Mind-Brain*. Cambridge, MA: The MIT Press, 1986.

Crane, Tim. *The Mechanical Mind: A Philosophical Introduction to Minds, Machines and Mental Representation*. 3rd ed. London; New York: Routledge, 2016.

Dreyfus, Hubert L. *What Computers Still Can't Do: The Limits of Artificial Intelligence*. Cambridge, MA: The MIT Press, 1992.

Nagel, T. "What is it like to be a bat?". *The Philosophical Review* 83 (1974): 435–450.

Pinker, Steven. *How the Mind Works*. New York: W.W. Norton & Company, 1997.

Ryle, Gilbert. *The Concept of Mind*. New York: Barnes & Noble Books, 1949.

Zahavi, Dan. *Phenomenology: The Basics*. New York: Routledge, 2019

Chapter 4: The Extended Mind

Clark, Andy. *Being There: Putting Brain, Body, and World Together Again*. Cambridge, MA: The MIT Press, 1997.

Clark, Andy. *Supersizing the Mind: Embodiment, Action, and Cognitive Extension*. New York: Oxford University Press, 2008.

Clark, Andy, and David Chalmers. "The extended mind." *Analysis* 58, no. 1 (1998): 7–19.

Sutton, John. "Extended cognition." In *The Stanford Encyclopedia of Philosophy*. Edited by Edward N. Zalta, Spring 2019. https://plato.stanford.edu/archives/spr2019/entries/extended-cognition/

Wilson, Robert A., and Lucia Foglia. "Embodied cognition." In *The Stanford Encyclopedia of Philosophy*. Edited by Edward N. Zalta, Fall 2017. https://plato.stanford.edu/archives/fall2017/entries/embodied-cognition/

Chapter 5: Interlude

Gallagher, Shaun. "The extended mind: State of the question." *The Southern Journal of Philosophy* 56, no. 4 (2018): 421–447.

Kaplan, D. M. "How to demarcate the boundaries of cognition." *Biology & Philosophy* 27, no. 4 (2012): 545–570.

Lassiter, C. and Vukov, J. "New ontological foundations for extended minds: Causal powers realism." *Phenomenology and the Cognitive Sciences* 23 (2024): 777–795.

Sterelny, K. "Minds: extended or scaffolded?" *Phenomenology and the Cognitive Sciences* 9 (2010): 465–481.

Chapter 6: Interpretations of the Extended Mind

Adams, Frederick, and Kenneth Aizawa. *The Bounds of Cognition*. Oxford; Malden, MA: Blackwell Publishing, 2008.

Anderson, Michael L. "Embodied cognition: A field guide." *Artificial Intelligence* 149, no. 1 (2003): 91–130.
Menary, Richard, ed. *The Extended Mind*. Cambridge, MA: The MIT Press, 2010.
Ward, Dave, and Mog Stapleton. "Es are good: Cognition as enacted, embodied, embedded, affective and extended." In *Consciousness in Interaction: The Role of the Natural and Social Context in Shaping Consciousness*. Edited by Fabio Paglieri. Amsterdam: John Benjamin Publishing Company, 2012.
Wilson, Margaret. "Six views of embodied cognition." *Psychonomic Bulletin & Review* 9, no. 4 (2002): 625–636.

Chapter 7: Weak Embodied Cognition

Adams, Fred. "Rehashing embodied cognition and the neural reuse hypothesis." *Synthese* 195, no. 1 (2018): 129–147.
Alsmith, Adrian, and Frédérique de Vignemont. "Embodying the mind and representing the body." *Mind & Language* 31, no. 3 (2016): 331–349.
Anderson, Michael L. *After Phrenology: Neural Reuse and the Interactive Brain*. Cambridge, MA: The MIT Press, 2014.
Barsalou, L. W. "Grounded cognition." *Annual Review of Psychology* 59 (2008): 617–645.
Damasio, Antonio. *Descartes' Error: Emotion, Reason, and the Human Brain*. New York: G.P. Putnam's Sons, 1994.
De Sousa, Ronald. *The Rationality of Emotion*. Cambridge, MA: The MIT Press, 1990.
Goldman, Alvin I. "A moderate approach to embodied cognitive science." *Review of Philosophy and Psychology* 2, no. 3 (2011): 555–569.
Paul, Annie Murphy. *The Extended Mind: The Power of Thinking Outside the Brain*. New York: Houghton Mifflin Harcourt Publishing Company, 2021.

Chapter 8: Objections to weak embodiment

Kagan, Aaron. "An enactive theory of emotion." *ETD Collection for Fordham University*, January 1, 2017, 1–266.
Kiverstein, Julian. "Embodied cognition and the neural reuse hypothesis." *Philosophical Psychology* 29, no. 3 (2016): 412–430.
Leslie, Sarah-Jane, Simon Cullen, and Adam J. Lerner, eds. *Current Controversies in Philosophy of Cognitive Science*. New York: Routledge, 2020.
Wittgenstein, Ludwig. *Philosophical Investigations*. New York: Wiley-Blackwell, 1953.

Chapter 9: Strong Embodiment

Chemero, Anthony. *Radically Embodied Cognitive Science*. Cambridge, MA: The MIT Press, 2009.
Di Paolo, Ezequiel A., Elena Clare Cuffari, and Hanne De Jaegher. *Linguistic Bodies: The Continuity between Life and Language*. Cambridge, MA: The MIT Press, 2018.
Gallagher, Shaun. *How the Body Shapes the Mind*. New York: Oxford University Press, 2005.

Maiese, Michelle. *Embodiment, Emotion, and Cognition*. New York: Palgrave Macmillan, 2011.
Noë, Alva. *Action in Perception*. Cambridge, MA: The MIT Press, 2004.
Thompson, Evan. *Mind in Life: Biology, Phenomenology, and the Sciences of Mind*. Cambridge, MA: The Belknap Press of Harvard University Press, 2007.
Varela, Francisco, Evan Thompson, and Eleanor Rosch. *The Embodied Mind: Cognitive Science and Human Experience*, revised edition. Cambridge, MA: The MIT Press, 2016.
Young, Iris Marion. "Throwing like a girl: A phenomenology of feminine body comportment motility and spatiality." *Human Studies* 3, no. 1 (1980): 137–156.

Chapter 10: Objections to Strong Embodiment

Block, Ned. "Review of Alva Noë, Action in perception." In *Consciousness, Function, and Representation, Volume 1: Collected Papers*. Cambridge, MA: The MIT Press, 2007, 363–378.
Clark, Andy, and Toribio, Mark. "Doing without representing?" *Synthese*, 101 (1994): 401–431.
Fodor, Jerry. "Where is my mind?" *London Review of Books* 31, no. 3 (2009): 13–15.
Goldinger, S. D., Papesh, M. H., Barnhart, A. S., Hansen, W. A., and Hout, M. C. "The poverty of embodied cognition." *Psychonomic Bulletin & Review* 23, no. 4 (2016): 959–978.

Chapter 11: Interlude: Exposition to Application

Lakoff, George, and Johnson, Mark. *Metaphors We Live By*. Chicago: University of Chicago Press, 1980.
Rosch, Eleanor. "Introduction to the revised edition." In *The Embodied Mind: Cognitive Science and Human Experience*. Edited by F. Varela, E. Thompson, and E. Rosch. Revised edition. Cambridge, MA: The MIT Press, 2016, xxxv–lv.
Sprevak, M. "Inference to the hypothesis of extended cognition." *Studies in History and Philosophy of Science, Part A* 41, no. 4 (2010): 353–362.
Thompson, Evan. "Introduction to the revised edition." In *The Embodied Mind: Cognitive Science and Human Experience*. Edited by F. Varela, E. Thompson, and E. Rosch. Revised edition. Cambridge, MA: The MIT Press, 2016: xvii–xxxiii.

Chapter 12: Free will, determinism, and embodiment

Frankfurt, Harry G. "Freedom of the will and the concept of a person." *The Journal of Philosophy* 68, no. 1 (1971): 5–20.
Kane, Robert. *A Contemporary Introduction to Free Will*. New York: Oxford University Press, 2005.
Mackenzie, Catriona, "Relational autonomy." In *The Oxford Handbook of Feminist Philosophy*. Edited by Kim Q. Hall and Ásta. New York: Oxford University Press, 2021: 374–384.

Strawson, P. F. "Freedom and resentment." In *Freedom and Resentment and Other Essays*. Routledge, 2008, 186–195. (Originally published in 1974.).
Wolf, Susan, "Sanity and the metaphysics of responsibility." In *Responsibility, Character and the Emotions: New Essays in Moral Psychology*. Edited by Ferdinand Schoeman. New York: Cambridge University Press, 1988, 46–62.

Chapter 13: Ethics and Embodiment

Churchland, Patricia S. *Braintrust: What Neuroscience Tells Us about Morality*. Princeton, NJ: Princeton University Press, 2011.
Gilligan, Carol. *In a Different Voice: Psychological Theory and Women's Development*. Cambridge, MA: Harvard University Press, 1993.
Prinz, Jesse. *The Emotional Construction of Morals*. New York: Oxford University Press, 2007.
Sander-Staudt, Maureen. "Care ethics." In *Internet Encyclopedia of Philosophy*. https://iep.utm.edu/care-ethics/
Sterba, James P. (Ed.). *Ethics: Classical Western Texts in Feminist and Multicultural Perspectives*. New York: Oxford University Press, 2000.

Chapter 14: Technology and Embodiment

Clark, Andy. *Natural-Born Cyborgs: Minds, Technologies, and the Future of Human Intelligence*. New York: Oxford University Press, 2003.
Heersmink, Richard. "The internet, cognitive enhancement, and the values of cognition." *Minds and Machines* 26, no. 4 (2016): 389–407.
Smart, Paul, Richard Heersmink, and Robert W. Clowes. "The cognitive ecology of the internet." In *Cognition Beyond the Brain: Computation, Interactivity and Human Artifice*. Edited by Stephen J. Cowley and Frédéric Vallée-Tourangeau. Springer International Publishing, 2017.

Chapter 15: Future Directions

Colombetti, Giovanna "Psychopathology and the enactive mind." In *The Oxford Handbook of Philosophy and Psychiatry*. Edited by K. W. M. Fulford, Martin Davies, Richard Gipps, George Graham, John Sadler, Giovanni Stanghellini, and Tim Thornton. Oxford: Oxford University Press, 2013, 1083–1102.
Gelfand, Michele. *Rule Makers, Rule Breakers: Tight and Loose Cultures and the Secret Signals that Direct our Lives*. New York: Scribner, 2018.
Henrich, Joseph. *The WEIRDest People in the World: How the West Became Psychologically Peculiar and Particularly Prosperous*. New York: Picador, 2020.
Nisbett, Richard. *The Geography of Thought: How Westerners and Asians Think Differently....and Why*. New York: Free Press, 2004.
Ratcliffe, Matthew. *Experiences of Depression: A Study in Phenomenology*. New York: Oxford University Press, 2014.
van der Kolk, Besser. *The Body Keeps the Score: Brain, Mind, and Body in the Healing of Trauma*. New York: Penguin Books, 2015.

GLOSSARY

Action-Oriented Representation A form of representation that directly guides an organism's actions in the world rather than passively mirroring external reality. For example, seeing a door handle as "graspable" is less about forming a detailed image of it and more about preparing the body to act on it.

Affordances Opportunities for action that the environment offers to an organism. A chair affords sitting, a staircase affords climbing, and a ripe fruit affords eating. James Gibson introduced this concept in ecological psychology to highlight that perception is about possibilities for action, not just the passive reception of stimuli.

Al-Kindi A 9th-century philosopher in the Islamic tradition, sometimes called "the Philosopher of the Arabs." He helped introduce and interpret Greek philosophy, especially Aristotle, for Arabic readers. Al-Kindi argued for the immateriality of the soul and saw philosophy and faith as compatible paths to truth.

Alan Turing British mathematician, logician, and computer scientist, often considered a founder of artificial intelligence. His 1950 paper proposed the "Turing Test" as a way to ask whether a machine could convincingly imitate human conversation.

American Pragmatism A philosophical movement developed in the late 19th and early 20th centuries by figures such as Charles Sanders Peirce, William James, and John Dewey (among others). It emphasizes the practical consequences of ideas, holding that beliefs gain meaning through their role in guiding action. Pragmatism blurs theory and practice, asking what difference a concept makes in lived experience.

Amodal Refers to representations not tied to any single sensory modality. For example, the concept of a triangle can be grasped through vision, touch, or language, but the abstract idea itself is amodal. Such representations highlight how cognition often transcends specific sensory channels.

Aristotle Ancient Greek philosopher, student of Plato, and tutor to Alexander the Great. Aristotle's writings cover nearly every area of philosophy, including metaphysics, logic, ethics, and psychology. His theory of the soul and his account of causation shaped centuries of debate in philosophy and science.

Atomism In philosophy of mind, atomism (distinct from ancient Greek atomism) holds that thoughts do not derive their contents from their connections with other thoughts. Your "cat" thoughts do not depend on "dog" or "mammal" thoughts in order to be about cats.

Autonomy The capacity to govern oneself and act in accordance with one's own principles or reasons. Philosophers debate whether autonomy requires strict independence or can also include relational support. In ethics and political thought, autonomy is tied to freedom, rights, and dignity.

Autonomy of Psychology The claim that psychology can explain mental phenomena without being reduced to neuroscience or biology. Proponents argue that concepts such as belief, intention, or desire operate at a different explanatory level than neural events. This view preserves psychology as an autonomous science of the mind.

Autopoietic Enactivism A form of enactivism influenced by Maturana and Varela's concept of autopoiesis, or self-production. On this view, organisms are self-maintaining systems that sustain their own identity through interactions with the environment. Cognition itself is understood as part of this ongoing process of self-organization.

Behaviorism A 20th-century psychological movement that explained behavior in terms of observable stimuli and responses. Rejecting appeals to hidden mental states, figures like Watson and Skinner studied learning and conditioning through controlled experiments. Though largely replaced by cognitive psychology, behaviorism shaped experimental methods and theories of learning.

Bodily Formats Ways the body itself represents or structures information, such as posture, gesture, or muscle tension. These bodily forms carry cognitive significance, linking action with thought. They remind us that not all representation is abstract or symbolic—some is built into bodily capacities.

Bridge Laws Claims that connect the laws of one scientific discipline with the laws of another. In the context of philosophy of mind, bridge laws, in principle, connect the laws of psychology with the laws of biology.

Brute Fact A fact that has no deeper explanation and simply "just is." Some philosophers suggest that the existence of the universe may be a brute fact. Others argue that consciousness itself could be such a fact if it resists reduction to more basic explanations.

B.F. Skinner American psychologist and one of the leading behaviorists. He developed the theory of operant conditioning, in which behavior is shaped by reinforcement and punishment. Skinner also explored how his theories might be applied to education, society, and debates about free will.

Carol Gilligan Psychologist and ethicist best known for her critique of Lawrence Kohlberg's stage theory of moral development. In *In a Different Voice* (1982), she argued that moral reasoning often emphasizes care, relationships, and responsibility, not just justice and rules. Her work founded an influential tradition of care ethics.

Categorical Imperative Immanuel Kant's central moral principle: act only on maxims you could will to be universal laws. Unlike hypothetical imperatives, which are conditional on desires, the categorical imperative applies unconditionally. It provides a test for whether an action is morally permissible. It entails treating agents as ends and never as means to an end.

Category Mistake A logical error in which something is presented as belonging to a category it cannot belong to. Gilbert Ryle used the example of someone visiting a university, seeing its buildings, and then asking "but where is the university?" Such mistakes reveal confusion in how concepts are applied.

Causal-informational theory of mental content A theory about how our thoughts get to have their contents. Our thoughts have the contents that they have because they carry information about the world that is reliably caused by some set of biological and/or cognitive mechanisms.

Character A person's relatively stable set of traits, habits, and dispositions that shape how they act and react. Philosophers since Aristotle have stressed the role of character in ethics, seeing virtues and vices as enduring qualities. Modern psychology also studies character in terms of personality and development.

Classical Compatibilism The view, often associated with Thomas Hobbes and David Hume, that freedom of the will and determinism are compatible. On this account, freedom means the ability to act according to one's desires without external constraint, even if those desires are themselves determined.

Cognitive Neuroscience An interdisciplinary field combining neuroscience and psychology to study the neural bases of cognition. It uses tools such as brain imaging, neuropsychological testing, and computational modeling. Cognitive neuroscience investigates how brain structures and processes underlie perception, memory, language, and decision-making.

Cognitive Revolution A mid-20th-century movement in psychology that rejected behaviorism and reintroduced the study of internal mental processes. Sparked by figures like Noam Chomsky and George Miller, it brought ideas from linguistics, computer science, and neuroscience into psychology. This "revolution" laid the foundations of modern cognitive science.

Collectivism A cultural orientation that prioritizes group goals, identity, and solidarity over individual interests. Collectivist cultures emphasize interdependence and duty to the community. It is often contrasted with individualism in psychology and social theory.

Complementarity Principle A view associated with second-wave extended mind. This principle holds that external resources that mesh with our onboard resources are part of the extended cognitive system. This is distinct from—though not inconsistent with—the Parity Principle.

Compatibilism The philosophical view that free will can coexist with determinism. Compatibilists argue that what matters for freedom is not the absence of causal determination but the ability to act in accordance with one's own reasons and desires. This position remains one of the dominant approaches in contemporary debates about responsibility.

Computational Theory of Mind The idea that cognitive processes are best understood as forms of computation. On this account, mental states are like symbolic representations, and the mind manipulates these according to rules, much like a computer running a program. The theory has been central to cognitive science since the mid-20th century.

Conceptual Metaphor Theory The idea that thought and language are largely structured by metaphors that we might not even notice. For example, the metaphor "time is money" shapes how we talk about and experience time (we can "save" time, "spend" time, or "waste" time). This theory suggests that our physical experiences help form these metaphorical concepts.

Conditional Argument A logical form used to support conditional claims. Conditional Arguments begin by assuming the antecedent (the part after the "if") and then deriving the consequent (the part after the "then").

Connectionism An approach in cognitive science that models the mind using artificial neural networks. Instead of symbol manipulation, cognition is seen as emerging from patterns of activation across interconnected nodes. Connectionism provides a contrast to classical computational models and has influenced psychology, neuroscience, and machine learning.

Conservatism in Science The idea that scientific communities tend to preserve established theories and resist change unless there is overwhelming evidence to shift consensus. This conservatism can protect against fads and premature conclusions but can also delay the acceptance of revolutionary ideas.

Content The meaning of a mental representation that is carried by the vehicle. The content of the thought "grass is green" is that *grass is green*. It's helpful to think of mental contents as being like the meaning of a sentence.

Content Externalism The thesis that the contents of our thoughts depend partly on features of our external environment. For example, the word "water" refers to H_2O in our world, but to "twin-water" (XYZ) in a hypothetical Twin Earth. Hilary Putnam used this thought experiment to argue that "meaning ain't just in the head."

Content Internalism The opposing view to externalism, holding that the content of our thoughts depends only on our internal mental states. On this picture, what you mean or think is determined by your cognitive structures alone, not by the external world. The debate between internalism and externalism shapes discussions in semantics and philosophy of mind.

Contradictions A situation in which two statements are in conflict with each other. For example, the statement "It is raining" and "It is not raining" cannot both be true at the same time. A contradiction always false. A contradiction is the opposite of a tautology.

Contrapositive In logic, the contrapositive of a conditional statement is formed by negating and reversing its terms. From "If P then Q," the contrapositive is "If not Q, then not P." Importantly, a conditional statement and its contrapositive are logically equivalent, a fact often used in arguments.

Cybernetics An interdisciplinary field studying systems of communication and control in animals, humans, and machines. Pioneered by Norbert Wiener, cybernetics introduced concepts like feedback loops that influenced robotics, biology, and cognitive science. It was a precursor to many contemporary ideas about self-regulating and adaptive systems.

Daoism The Dao is a cosmic force. Daoists hold that people can achieve a state of peace and balance by embracing key principles such as *wu wei* (effortless action or non-interference), simplicity, and the dynamic balance of *yin and yang*.

David Hume An 18th-century Scottish philosopher known for his empiricism and skepticism. Hume argued that our belief in causation is a product of habit, not rational proof, and he raised the famous "is–ought" problem about deriving moral claims from facts.

David Lewis A 20th-century philosopher who made major contributions to philosophy of mind, particularly functionalism and theories of mental content. He argued that qualitative aspects of experience are a kind of practical knowledge.

David Marr A cognitive scientist who proposed a highly influential framework for analyzing cognitive systems at three levels—computational (what the system does), algorithmic (how it does it), and implementational (what physical structures realize it).

Determinism The philosophical view that for every event, including human action, there are conditions that could cause no other event. This means that all events are completely determined by preceding causes and the laws of nature. This view is often contrasted with libertarianism.

Direct Perception In ecological psychology, the view that perception picks up information directly from the environment, without needing mental reconstruction or inference. For example, when you see a chair, you directly perceive its affordance for sitting. This challenges views that perception is mediated by internal representations.

Disembodiment/Disembodied The traditional view that the mind and body are distinct and separate substances. The body is often seen as a temporary home or vessel for the mind. In weaker forms, it holds that minds and bodies are the same kind of substance but that they can be scientifically studied independently of each other.

Distal Causes Causes that are removed in time or space from their effects. For instance, a genetic mutation might be a distal cause of a disease that only manifests decades later. Distal causes are often contrasted with proximal causes, which are immediate and direct.

Double-Sensation A concept from the phenomenology of touch. When you touch one hand with the other, you experience both being touched and touching. This "double-sensation" illustrates how bodily experience reveals the intertwining of subject and object.

Ecological Psychology An approach to psychology pioneered by James Gibson. It emphasizes the mutual relationship between organism and environment, particularly how animals directly perceive affordances for action. Ecological psychology resists seeing perception as merely the internal processing of sensory data.

Edmund Husserl A German philosopher and founder of phenomenology. Husserl sought to carefully describe the structures of lived experience, bracketing assumptions about the external world. His work influenced Heidegger, Merleau-Ponty, and many others in 20th-century philosophy.

Efficient Causation One of Aristotle's four causes, referring to the agent or process that produces an effect. For example, a sculptor is the efficient cause of a statue.

Eliminativist A person who believes that a certain category of things does not exist. In philosophy of mind, an eliminativist might argue that concepts like "beliefs" or "desires" are just fictions and won't be part of a complete scientific description of the mind.

Elizabeth Anscombe A 20th-century British philosopher best known for her work on action theory and intention. Anscombe argues that intentional actions are those to which a specific kind of "Why?" question is applicable, where the answer gives the agent's reason for acting. This reason isn't a cause, but rather an explanation that places the action within a larger context of the agent's goals and purposes.

Embodied The view that our minds are shaped by the structure and function of our bodies. This perspective argues that thinking doesn't just happen "in our heads," but that the body plays a key role in how we think, feel, and experience the world.

Empathy The capacity to understand and share the feelings of another person. Empathy plays an important role in ethics, psychology, and philosophy of mind. Some philosophers distinguish between affective empathy (feeling with another) and cognitive empathy (understanding another's perspective).

Enactive A perspective that emphasizes that cognition is a process of active, sensory-motor engagement with the world. The mind isn't just reacting to the environment; it's co-creating meaning with it through our actions.

Enactivism A theory of mind that emphasizes that cognition is a process of active, sensory-motor engagement with the world and that cognition arises through dynamic interactions between an organism and its environment. On this view, perception and action are inseparable—we make sense of the world by engaging with it. Enactivism is often contrasted with representational theories of cognition.

Epistemology A major branch of philosophy that studies knowledge. It explores questions like: What is knowledge? How do we get it? How do we know if we have it?

Extended Mind/Extended Mind Hypothesis The idea that the mind and its cognitive processes are not contained solely within the skull but can extend out into the world to include the body and even external tools and environments like a smartphone or a notebook. Clark and Chalmers (1998) used the case of Otto's notebook to argue that if an external object functions like memory and is reliably used, it counts as part of the mind. The hypothesis sparked ongoing debates about the boundaries of cognition.

Franz Brentano A 19th-century philosopher who argued that intentionality—the quality of being about something—is the defining feature of the mental. Brentano's lectures influenced many later thinkers, including Husserl, Meinong, and Freud. His work helped set the stage for phenomenology and psychology.

Freedom of Action The ability to choose an action from a range of possibilities without being physically coerced. For example, you have the freedom of action to either read this book or go outside for a walk.

Freedom of Opportunity The socially constrained or enabled possibility of performing some action, given that the agent has the freedom of action to do so. Freedoms of opportunity often connect with social and cultural constraints and conventions.

Freedom of Will A more profound concept than freedom of action. It is the ability to have willed otherwise—to have chosen a different course of action even if all the prior events leading up to your choice were exactly the same. It's the freedom to form the kinds of desires that motivate you to act.

Frontal Lobe The part of the brain associated with planning, reasoning, decision-making, and voluntary movement. Damage to the frontal lobe can result in changes to personality, impaired judgment, and difficulties with self-control. It plays a central role in higher-order cognitive functions.

Functionalism A theory in philosophy of mind that defines mental states by their functional roles rather than their physical makeup. For example, pain is what occurs when tissue damage causes a certain response, regardless of whether it is realized in neurons, silicon, or another medium. Functionalism allows for the possibility of machine or alien minds.

George Berkeley An 18th-century philosopher who argued for immaterialism, the view that reality consists only of minds and ideas. Berkeley's slogan was "to be is to be perceived," meaning objects exist only insofar as they are experienced by a mind. His work was both a response to materialism and an influence on later idealist traditions.

George Miller A psychologist best known for his 1956 paper "The Magical Number Seven, Plus or Minus Two," which argued that working memory has a limited capacity. Miller's work helped establish the importance of studying internal mental processes during the Cognitive Revolution. He was also a founder of cognitive psychology as a field.

Gestalt Psychology A school of psychology that emerged in early 20th-century Germany, emphasizing holistic perception. Gestalt theorists argued that "the whole is greater than the sum of its parts," highlighting principles like figure-ground organization and perceptual grouping. Their work challenged reductionist approaches to perception.

Gilbert Ryle A 20th-century philosopher best known for his critique of Cartesian dualism. In *The Concept of Mind* (1949), he described the mind–body split as a "category mistake." Ryle argued that mental terms should be understood as ways of talking about behavior and dispositions rather than inner, ghostly processes.

Gottlob Frege A 19th-century German logician and philosopher who revolutionized logic and semantics. He distinguished between the sense (*Sinn*) and reference (*Bedeutung*) of terms, an idea that shaped the philosophy of language. Frege's formal logic laid the groundwork for analytic philosophy and influenced figures like Bertrand Russell and Ludwig Wittgenstein.

Hard Problem of Consciousness A term coined by David Chalmers to describe the difficulty of explaining why and how physical processes in the brain give rise to subjective experience. Unlike the "easy problems" of explaining functions such as attention or memory, the hard problem focuses on qualia, or the felt quality of experiences. The hard problem is considered "hard" because philosophers and scientists are not sure what an adequate theory of subjective experience would even look like.

High Relational Mobility Cultures Cultures where people have a lot of choice in their social relationships and have to actively work to form and maintain friendships. These cultures contrast with those where relationships are more fixed and stable.

Hilary Putnam A philosopher of mind and language who developed influential arguments for functionalism in the 1960s and 1970s. His "Twin Earth" thought experiment reshaped debates about meaning and reference by showing that the environment partly determines what our words mean. Later, he became a critic of functionalism and explored pragmatist approaches.

Holism The view that the meanings of our concepts are interconnected and shape one another. For example, the content of your "dog" thoughts is determined (at least in part) by other thoughts and concepts, like "wolf" or "fetch." It is contrasted with atomism.

Humberto Maturana A Chilean biologist and philosopher who, with Francisco Varela, developed the concept of autopoiesis, or self-production. Maturana's work emphasized that living systems are autonomous and self-maintaining. His ideas influenced enactivism, cognitive science, and systems theory.

Hypothetical Syllogism A deductive rule of inference following the pattern—if P, then Q; if Q, then R; therefore, if P, then R. For example, "If Homer loves donuts, then he will go to the donut shop. If Homer goes to the donut shop, he will be late for work. Therefore, if Homer loves donuts, he'll be late for work."

Identity *and* Individuation Conditions Criteria used to determine when an entity is the same over time and what distinguishes it from others.

For example, what makes a river "the same river" despite constant changes in water? These conditions are central in metaphysics, logic, and debates about personal identity.

Identity Theory *(aka mind-brain identity theory)* A theory in philosophy of mind. It says that mental states are identical to brain states in the way that Mark Twain is identical to Sam Clemens. Your belief that grass is green is identical to a state of your brain.

Immanent Causation A type of causation where the cause remains within the agent rather than acting externally. For example, a person initiating an action from within themselves is sometimes described as an immanent cause. This concept is contrasted with transeunt causation, where one thing causes changes in another.

Immanuel Kant An 18th-century philosopher whose *Critique of Pure Reason* reshaped metaphysics and epistemology. Kant argued that our minds actively structure experience through categories such as space and time. In ethics, he is known for the categorical imperative, a universal moral principle.

Incompatibilism The view that free will and determinism cannot both be true. If determinism is correct, incompatibilists argue, then every action is necessitated by prior events, leaving no room for genuine freedom. Libertarians about free will typically hold this position.

Individualism A cultural orientation that emphasizes personal independence, self-reliance, and individual goals over group commitments. Individualist cultures value autonomy and self-expression. It is often contrasted with collectivism.

Individualistic Autonomy A conception of autonomy that stresses independence from others. On this view, being autonomous means being free of outside interference or social influence. Critics argue this overlooks the relational and social dimensions of human life.

Indirect Perception The view that perception is mediated by internal representations or processing, rather than being direct. For example, when we see an object, our brains may construct a representation of it from sensory input before we consciously experience it. This view contrasts with direct perception theories.

Inference to the Best Explanation A form of reasoning where one infers that the hypothesis which best explains the available evidence is likely to be true. For example, if footprints are found in the snow, the best explanation may be that someone walked there. This type of reasoning is widely used in science and philosophy.

Infinite Regress A problem that arises when an explanation requires an endless chain of further explanations. For example, if perception is like a picture in the head, then there must be "someone"—a homunculus—inside the head viewing the picture. But then that homunculus must itself have another homunculus inside *its* head to explain how it can perceive the "picture" in the head.

Intentionality The "aboutness" of our thoughts. It is the unique property of mental states like beliefs, desires, and intentions to be directed at or to be about objects and states of affairs in the world.

Intersubjective Refers to what is shared or accessible between different subjects or perspectives. Intersubjectivity often describes how meaning, norms, or experiences can be mutually recognized. It contrasts with what is merely subjective or purely private.

Jakob von Uexküll A biologist and philosopher who introduced the concept of the *Umwelt*, or the subjective world each organism inhabits. He emphasized that perception and meaning are species-specific, shaped by an organism's sensory and motor capacities. His work influenced phenomenology, semiotics, and ecological psychology.

James Gibson A psychologist who developed ecological psychology and the concept of affordances. Gibson argued that perception is direct—organisms detect information in the environment that specifies possibilities for action. His work reshaped how psychology understands vision and action.

Jerry Fodor A philosopher of mind and cognitive scientist who argued for modularity in the mind, suggesting that certain cognitive processes are domain-specific and encapsulated. He also proposed the "language of thought hypothesis," which claims that thinking occurs in a mental code with syntax and semantics. Fodor's ideas were central to cognitive science in the late 20th century.

John Stuart Mill A 19th-century philosopher and economist who defended utilitarianism and liberal political thought. In ethics, Mill refined Bentham's utilitarianism by distinguishing higher and lower pleasures. His writings on liberty and individuality remain influential in political philosophy.

Know-how A type of practical knowledge or skill. It is the ability to do something, like knowing how to ride a bicycle or play the piano, and it's often difficult to put into words.

Know-that A type of propositional knowledge or factual knowledge. It is the knowledge of a proposition, such as knowing that the sky is blue or that the Earth revolves around the sun.

Körper A German word for the body as a physical, biological object of scientific or medical study. It is the body viewed from a third-person, objective perspective, often contrasted with Leib or the "lived body."

Lawrence Kohlberg A psychologist known for his stage theory of moral development. Kohlberg proposed that individuals progress through stages of moral reasoning, from obedience to universal ethical principles. His work inspired both followers and critics, including Carol Gilligan.

Leib A German word for the "lived body"—the body as we subjectively experience it. It is the body as a part of our conscious experience, from a first-person perspective.

Libertarianism The philosophical view that we are free and our choices are not determined by prior causes. A libertarian believes in the reality of freedom of will.

Limit Cases Situations at the boundaries of concepts or theories that test their adequacy. For example, thought experiments often rely on limit cases to probe the meaning of "mind" or "person." They help clarify how far a theory can be stretched before it breaks down.

Localization The idea that specific functions in the brain are tied to particular regions. For example, Broca's area is linked to speech production. While neuroscience has supported many cases of localization, debates remain about how modular or distributed brain functions truly are.

Ludwig Wittgenstein A 20th-century philosopher who made groundbreaking contributions in two phases. In the *Tractatus Logico-Philosophicus*, he developed a picture theory of language. Later, in *Philosophical Investigations*, he emphasized language games and the social nature of meaning. Wittgenstein's work has deeply influenced philosophy of language and mind.

Male Gaze A concept from feminist theory, especially in film criticism, describing how women are often depicted from a heterosexual male perspective. This "gaze" objectifies women and reinforces gendered power relations. The idea has been expanded into broader critiques of social representation and social norms.

Mental Representations Internal structures or states that stand for things in the world. Representations can be images, symbols, or concepts used in reasoning, perception, and memory. The idea is central in cognitive science and philosophy of mind, though it is contested by non-representational theories of cognition.

Mentalese Another name for the language supposed in the Language of Thought Hypothesis. This is the innate language all humans are born with and which is mapped onto natural languages (like English or Urdu).

Metaethics The branch of ethics that examines the status, foundations, and meaning of moral judgments. It asks questions such as: Are moral claims objective or subjective? Are they true or false, or do they merely express emotions? Metaethics provides the conceptual backdrop for normative and applied ethics.

Mind over matter The popular idea that through mental activity, you can exert control and overcome bodily or physical limitations.

Modality Refers to the different sensory channels or ways of perceiving the world, such as vision, hearing, touch, taste, and smell. Philosophers and psychologists study how modalities integrate and interact in experience.

Modularity The theory that the mind is made up of specialized subsystems or "modules" for different tasks. Jerry Fodor's modularity hypothesis argued that modules are domain-specific, fast, and encapsulated. The extent of modularity remains debated in cognitive science and neuroscience.

Modus Ponens A deductive rule of inference following the pattern—if P, then Q; P; therefore, Q. For example, "If Homer loves donuts, then he will go to the donut shop. Homer loves donuts. Therefore, he will go to the donut shop."

Modus Tollens A deductive rule of inference following the pattern—if P, then Q; not-Q; therefore, not-P. For example, "If Homer likes going to work, then he arrives early. Homer does not arrive early. Therefore, Homer does not like going to work."

Motor Cortex A region of the brain responsible for planning, controlling, and executing voluntary movements. It is organized somatotopically, meaning different parts correspond to different body regions. Damage to the motor cortex can impair motor control and coordination.

Multiple Realization The idea that mental states can be realized in different physical substrates. For example, pain could be realized in human neural activity, but also in alien biochemistry or computer circuits. This view challenges reductive physicalism by showing that higher-level states can have diverse physical bases.

Natural Meaning A distinction made by philosopher Paul Grice. Natural meaning occurs when something inherently signifies something else, such as dark clouds meaning rain or smoke meaning fire. This is contrasted with non-natural meaning, which involves human intentions and communication.

Necessary Condition A condition that must be met in order for the statement to be true. For example, having a driver's license is a necessary condition for (legally) driving a car. These are contrasted with sufficient conditions.

Ned Block A philosopher of mind known for his work on consciousness and critiques of functionalism. Block introduced the "China brain" thought experiment to challenge whether functionalist accounts can capture subjective experience. He also distinguished between access consciousness and phenomenal consciousness.

Nelson Goodman An American philosopher (1906-1998). One of his most well-known contributions is the "new riddle of induction," though he also contributed to discussions of reflective equilibrium.

Neural Reuse The idea that neural circuits originally evolved for one purpose can be reused for others. For example, brain areas involved in motor control may also support abstract reasoning. Neural reuse highlights the brain's plasticity and efficiency.

Neurath's Boat A metaphor by philosopher Otto Neurath for the scientific enterprise. We are like sailors rebuilding a ship at sea—we must repair and replace planks while staying afloat. This illustrates the idea that science is a continuous process without an ultimate foundation.

Noam Chomsky A linguist who revolutionized the study of language with his theory of generative grammar. Chomsky argued that humans have an innate "universal grammar" that explains language acquisition despite limited input, leading to the "poverty of the stimulus" argument. His work helped launch the Cognitive Revolution.

Normative Refers to what ought to be, as opposed to what is. Normative claims set standards for judgment, whether in ethics, epistemology, or social practice. For example, "You should keep your promises" is a normative statement.

Objective Refers to what is independent of individual perspective or opinion. Objective truths are taken to hold regardless of who perceives them, such as the laws of mathematics or physics. In contrast, subjective claims vary with personal viewpoints.

Operant Learning A form of learning studied by B.F. Skinner in which behavior is shaped by reinforcement and punishment. For example, a child may learn to say "please" if it reliably leads to a reward. Operant learning remains central in psychology and behavior analysis.

Optic Flow The pattern of visual motion experienced as an observer moves through an environment. Optic flow provides information about speed, direction, and obstacles. James Gibson highlighted its importance for understanding perception and navigation.

Panpsychism The view that consciousness is a fundamental and ubiquitous feature of the universe. According to panpsychism, even basic physical entities may have some form of experience. Though controversial, it has been defended as a way to bridge the gap between matter and mind.

Parity Principle Introduced by Clark and Chalmers in their defense of the extended mind. The principle states that if an external process functions like an internal cognitive process and is reliably available, it is part of the mind. This challenges traditional boundaries between mind and world.

Participatory Sense-Making A concept from enactive and social cognition theories. It describes how meaning emerges through interaction between agents, rather than being generated solely by individuals. In this view, understanding and coordination are co-created in social encounters.

Paul Grice A philosopher of language known for his theory of conversational implicature. Grice distinguished between natural meaning (like smoke meaning fire) and non-natural meaning (where a speaker intends to communicate something). His Cooperative Principle remains foundational in pragmatics.

Peter Strawson A 20th-century philosopher who contributed to metaphysics and philosophy of language. In *Individuals* (1959), he explored issues of identity and individuation. He also emphasized the importance of "reactive attitudes" in understanding moral responsibility.

Phenomenology A philosophical movement founded by Edmund Husserl, focused on describing the structures of experience. Phenomenologists study how things appear in consciousness, setting aside assumptions about external reality. Later figures like Heidegger and Merleau-Ponty developed phenomenology into existential and embodied directions.

Physicalism The metaphysical thesis that everything is physical, or at least dependent on physical facts. Physicalists argue that mental states are ultimately physical states.

Pierre Laplace An 18th–19th-century French mathematician and philosopher who defended a deterministic view of the universe. Laplace famously imagined a vast intellect (Laplace's Demon) that, knowing all physical facts, could predict the future with certainty. His ideas influenced debates on determinism and predictability.

Poverty of the Stimulus A term from Chomskyan linguistics. It refers to the idea that the linguistic input children receive is too limited to account for their rapid and uniform language acquisition. This supports the claim that humans possess innate linguistic structures.

Practical Knowledge Know-how: Knowledge that is tied to doing rather than abstract representation. For example, knowing how to ride a bike or play an instrument involves practical knowledge. This is distinct from propositional knowledge (know-that).

Practical Wisdom Aristotle's concept of *phronesis*, the ability to deliberate well about how to act in particular situations. Practical wisdom involves not just general rules but sensitivity to context and experience. It is central in virtue ethics.

Primary Intersubjectivity A term from developmental psychology and phenomenology referring to the pre-reflective, embodied sharing between infants and caregivers. Before language, infants engage in eye contact, mimicry, and emotional attunement. This early interaction grounds later social cognition.

Principle of Alternate Possibilities A principle in debates about free will stating that a person is morally responsible for what they have done only if they could have done otherwise. Harry Frankfurt famously challenged this principle with thought experiments, sparking ongoing debate.

Principle of Bivalence A fundamental logical principle that says that the only two truth-values are true and false.

Principle of Noncontradiction A fundamental logical principle stating that a statement cannot be both true and false at the same time and in the same respect.

Propositions Abstract, content-bearing entities that can be true or false. For example, the sentence "snow is white" expresses the proposition that snow is white. Philosophers debate whether propositions exist independently of language and what their ontological status is.

Proprioception The sense of the body's position and movement in space, often called the "sixth sense." Proprioception relies on receptors in muscles and joints. It allows coordination and balance without needing to look at one's own limbs.

Protention and Retention Terms from phenomenology describing how consciousness stretches over time. Retention is the holding of just-past experience (like the last note of a melody), while protention is the anticipation of what is about to come. Together they explain how we experience temporal continuity.

Psychological Determinism The view that human thoughts and actions are fully determined by psychological states such as desires, beliefs, and past experiences. This position raises questions about freedom and responsibility. It differs from physical determinism in focusing on mental rather than physical causes.

Qualia The subjective, qualitative aspects of experience, such as what it feels like to taste chocolate or see red. Qualia are often used in arguments against physicalism, as they seem resistant to purely physical explanation.

Question-Begging A logical fallacy in which the conclusion is assumed in the premises. For example, "Paranormal activity is real because I've experienced what can only be described as paranormal activity." Such reasoning offers no independent support for the conclusion.

Reflective Equilibrium A method in moral and political philosophy that involves going back and forth between general principles and particular judgments, making adjustments to each until they form a coherent and mutually supportive set of beliefs.

Relational Autonomy A conception of autonomy that emphasizes how self-determination is shaped by relationships and social context. For example, choosing freely often depends on supportive environments rather than pure independence. This view contrasts with individualistic autonomy.

Reliable Coupling A condition in extended cognition theories. It refers to when an agent and an external tool or process form a dependable system that supports cognition. For example, a person who consistently uses a notebook to extend memory exhibits reliable coupling.

Second-Order Desires A concept from Harry Frankfurt describing desires about one's desires. For example, wanting to quit smoking is a second-order desire about the first-order desire to smoke.

Second-Wave Extended Mind Refers to developments in extended mind theory after the original Clark and Chalmers paper. This wave emphasizes not only individual coupling with tools but also broader patterns of social, cultural, and technological scaffolding. It expands the scope of how cognition can be extended.

Sensorimotor Contingencies Regularities in how sensory input changes with movement. For example, turning your head alters the pattern of visual input in predictable ways. Enactivist and embodied theories argue that mastering these contingencies is central to perception.

Sense-Making The process by which organisms actively interpret and give meaning to their environment. In enactivism, sense-making is not just passive reception but involves valuing and responding to the world. It highlights the role of the organism's perspective in cognition.

Simulation Theory A theory of mindreading that holds that we understand others by simulating their mental states within ourselves. For instance, we may predict someone's action by imagining what we would do in their situation. Simulation theory contrasts with "theory theory," which emphasizes using folk-psychological rules.

Situationism A position in moral psychology that challenges the idea of stable character traits. Situationists argue that behavior is often more influenced by situational factors than by virtues or vices. This view has sparked debates with virtue ethics about the reality of character.

Social Affordances Opportunities for action offered by the social environment. For example, a smile affords approach and interaction, while a raised hand may afford cooperation or caution. Social affordances expand the Gibsonian concept into the interpersonal domain.

Soul The spiritual or immaterial part of a human being, often considered to be the seat of consciousness and personality.

Space of Possibilities The set of theories (or ideas) we are left with after considering a variety of combinations, typically based on principles of logic.

St. Augustine An early Christian philosopher whose writings shaped medieval thought. Augustine reflected deeply on memory, time, and the will. He developed Plato's dualism in the context of Christianity.

St. Thomas Aquinas Aquinas, drawing from Aristotle, believed that humans are a composite of a body and a soul, that we are ensouled bodies. In this view, the soul isn't a separate entity merely inhabiting the body, but rather the substantial form that gives the body life and defines it as a human being. The soul isn't a thing but an organizing principle. The body is the matter that the soul organizes.

Strong Embodiment A form of embodied cognition that claims the body and environment are absolutely essential and constitutive of the mind. In this view, the mind literally wouldn't be what it is without the body.

Subjective Refers to what is dependent on individual perspective or experience. For example, the taste of coffee may be pleasant for one person and unpleasant for another. Subjectivity contrasts with objectivity and intersubjectivity.

Sufficient Condition A condition that, if met, guarantees the truth of a statement. For example, being a square is a sufficient condition for being a rectangle. Philosophers contrast sufficient with necessary conditions in logical analysis.

Sui Generis A Latin phrase meaning "of its own kind" or unique. It is often used in philosophy to describe something that cannot be reduced to other categories, such as moral norms or certain social phenomena.

Tautology A claim that is always true, like "the cup weighs 4 ounces or it does not weigh 4 ounces." No matter how much the cup weighs, it is either 4 ounces or it isn't. A tautology is the opposite of a contradiction.

Theory of Mind The ability to attribute mental states like beliefs, desires, and intentions to oneself and others. Theory of mind allows us to predict and interpret behavior.

Theory Theory A view of mindreading that holds that we understand others by employing an implicit "theory" of how minds work. On this account, attributing beliefs and desires is like applying folk psychology. It contrasts with simulation theory.

Thick Concepts Concepts that combine descriptive and evaluative aspects. For example, calling an action "cruel" both describes it and evaluates it negatively. Thick concepts are debated in ethics because they blur the line between facts and values.

Thin Concepts Concepts in ethics that are primarily evaluative without much descriptive content, such as "good" or "bad." They contrast with thick concepts like "brave" or "selfish." Thin concepts are central in debates about moral language.

Thomas Hobbes A 17th-century philosopher best known for his political work *Leviathan*. Hobbes also contributed to philosophy of mind, describing thought as motion in the body. His mechanistic outlook influenced later materialist theories.

Thomas Reid An 18th-century philosopher and founder of the Scottish common sense school. Reid defended direct realism, the view that we perceive the world as it is, against skeptical and idealist arguments. His work was an alternative to Hume's empiricism.

Thought Experiment A hypothetical scenario used to test intuitions and clarify concepts. Famous examples include Descartes' evil demon or Putnam's Twin Earth. Thought experiments play a major role in philosophy of mind and cognitive science.

Transducer A device or mechanism that converts one form of energy or signal into another. In perception, sensory receptors act as transducers by converting physical stimuli (like light or sound) into neural signals.

Transeunt Causation Causation in which one entity brings about change in another. For example, a cue ball striking another ball is an instance of transeunt causation. It is contrasted with immanent causation, where the cause remains within the agent.

Turing Test Proposed by Alan Turing in 1950 as a way of asking whether a machine can "think." The test involves a machine's ability to carry on a conversation indistinguishable from that of a human.

Umwelt A German word meaning the "self-world." It refers to the world around an organism as it is subjectively experienced by that organism. Each species has its own unique *Umwelt* based on its sensory capabilities and needs.

Vehicles That which carries the content in a mental representation. One example is the Language of Thought, which says that the vehicles of thoughts are sentence-like entities.

Virtue A stable character trait or disposition to act well. For Aristotle, virtues like courage and temperance are cultivated through practice and lead to human flourishing. Virtue ethics emphasizes the role of such traits in moral life.

Weak Embodiment A form of embodied cognition that claims the body and environment inform the structure and content of our mental representations. On this view, the body and environment are important for understanding why we think and perceive as we do, but it retains some of the conceptual tools of disembodiment.

Will The capacity for deliberate action and decision. Philosophers debate whether the will is free or determined, and how it relates to desire and reason. Discussions of the will are central in ethics, metaphysics, and psychology.

William James An American philosopher and psychologist who pioneered pragmatism and functional psychology. James emphasized the fluid, stream-like nature of consciousness and the practical consequences of belief. His work bridged philosophy and early psychology.

Willard Van Orman Quine A 20th-century philosopher who challenged the analytic–synthetic distinction and argued for holism in language and science. Quine rejected the idea of a clear boundary between philosophy and empirical science. His work reshaped philosophy of language and epistemology.

Working Memory A system for temporarily holding and manipulating information needed for cognitive tasks like reasoning, comprehension, and problem-solving. Unlike long-term memory, working memory has a limited capacity. It is a central concept in psychology and neuroscience.

Zenon Pylyshyn A cognitive scientist and philosopher known for his defense of classical computational models of the mind. He argued that cognition is fundamentally symbolic and rule-governed.

INDEX

Pages in *italics* refer to figures, pages in ***bold-italics*** refer to boxes and pages in **bold** refer to tables and pages followed by n refer to notes.

action-oriented representation 44, 230
Adams, Fred 60–61, 100–110
affordances 118, 121–122, 127, 129, 138, 143, 214, 217, 230
Agency ch. 12 *passim*, 165, ***166***, 174, 205
Aizawa, Ken 60–61
Al-Kindi 20, 230
amodal representations 89–90, 97, 99, 104, 167, 231
Anscombe, Elizabeth ***146***, ***177***, 236
aporia 7–9, 51, 67, 70, 187
Aquinas, St. Thomas xii, 246
Aristotle x–xii, ***8***, 17, 46, 113, 213, 231–232, 247–248
atomism 104, 231, 238
Augustine, St. 20–***21***, 246
autonomy 172, ***173***, 176, 178, 179n9, 182–183, 186, 191, 205, 210, 231, 239
autonomy, individualistic 171
autonomy, relational 171, 245

behaviorism ***22***, 23, 81, 231, 233
Berkeley, George 237
Block, Ned 14, 68, 167, 242
bodily formats 86, 90, 95–96, 108, 231
Brain Meme *49*
Brentano, Franz 30, 237
bridge laws 12, 232
Broca, Paul ***62***, 92–93
brute fact 39, 232

care ethics 195–196, 198n24, 232
categorical imperative 183, 232, 239
category mistake 36, ***37***, 232, 238
causal-constitution fallacy 60–61, 70–71, 74
causal-informational theory of mental content 42–43, 232
causation, efficient ***160***, 236
Chalmers, David xi, ch. 4 *passim*, 47, 51, 61, 81, 220–221, 236, 238, 243
Chomsky, Noam ***23***, 97, 233, 243
Churchland, Patricia and Paul 13
Clark, Andy xi, ch. 4 *passim*, 72, 76, 85, 98, 146, 154, 188, 200–202, 211, 236, 243, 246
cognition, embedded 37, 77–78, 84n8, 152, 155, 173, 226
cognitive neuroscience 62, 143–145, 233
cognitive revolution 23–24, 29, 233
collectivism 217, 233
compatibilism 232–233

complementarity principle 74–76, 80, 233
computational theory of mind 25, 233
conceptual metaphor theory 90–92, 99, 105, 177, 215, 233
conditional argument 32, 233
connectionism ***29***, 233–234
conservatism in science ***87***, 143, 234
content externalism ***109***, 234
content internalism ***109***, 234
content, mental 26–29, 31, 42, 44, 232, 235
contradictions 7, ***8***, 234
contrapositive 187, 234
cybernetics 63n8, 234

Daoism ***8***, 234
Dennett, Daniel 15, ***26***, 61, 221
Descartes, René 20–22, 45n1–45n2, 63n2, ***87***, 89, 97, 159, 169, 238, 248
disembodiment x–xi, ch. 3 *passim*, 67, 80, **81**, 85, 100n1, 103, 106, 110, 133, 196, 214, 218n5, 235
double-sensation 35–36, 102, 235–236
Dreyfus, Hubert 174–175, 226

eliminativism 12–13, 15, 34, 58–59, ***87***, 198n21, 236
embodiment, strong xi, 77, 80, **81**, 82, 110, ch. 9 *passim*, ch. 10 *passim*, 177–178, 188–189, 191–193, 197, 207–208, 214, 216–217, 247
embodiment, weak xi, 70, 77, **81**, 82, ch. 7 *passim*, ch. 8 *passim*, 111, 117, 134, 152, 155, 166–168, 176–177, 185, 216, 248
emotion 19, 55, 85, 98, 131–133, 137–138, 191–192, 194, 198n16, 216
empathy 131, 193–194, 197, 218, 236
enactivism 79, 236, 238, 246
enactivism, autopoietic ***137***, 141n27, 231
enactivism, sensorimotor 123–126
Entscheidungsproblem 24
epistemic actions 79
epistemology ***80***, 197n12, 236, 239, 243, 249
extended mind hypothesis xi, 14, 45, chapter 4 *passim*, 67–69, chapter 6 *passim*, 85, 98–99, 100n9, 111, 152–153, 155n1, 188–189, 233, 236, 243, 246

Fodor, Jerry 16, 46n17, 88, 145, 221, 240
freedom of action 164–170, 174, 178, 237
freedom of opportunity 174, 178, 237
freedom of will 164–170, 174, 237, 241
functionalism 13–14, ***20***, 33, 55–56, 58–60, 64n21, 68, 98–99, 107–108, 167, 235, 237–238, 242

Gage, Phineas 61–62
Gallagher, Shaun xii, 144, 147, 221, 226–227
Gestalt psychology ***36***, 237
Gibson, J.J. xi, 121, 152, 221, 230, 235, 240, 243
Gilligan, Carol 195, 232, 241
Glenberg, Arthur 94–95, 221
Goldin-Meadow, Susan 80
Goldman, Alvin xi, 86–89, 92, 95–98, 101, 104–106, 216, 221
Goodman, Nelson 17n2, 222
Grice, Paul 38, 242, 244

hard problem of consciousness 40, 238
Heidegger, Martin 63n8, 212, 235, 244
Hobbes, Thomas 138, 232, 247
holism 104, 238, 249
Hume, David 98, 162, 177, 179n6, 197, 198n19, 232, 235
Husserl, Edmund ***35***, 117, 120, 134, 193, 212, 235, 237, 244

Ibn Sina 20, ***21***, 45n1
identity theory 12, 17n5, 26, 33–34, 58, 63n1, 194, 239
immanent causation 159, 239, 248
infinite regress ***26***, 39, 239
instrumentalism 15, 58–59, 64n20
intentionality 30–31, 118, 133–136, 141n25–141n26, 193, 237, 240

James, William 121, ***131***, 221, 248

Kant, Immanuel 45n2, ***172***, 182, 186, 197n1, 198n22, 218n4, 239
know-how 79, ***80***, 209–210, 240, 244

know-that *80*, 240, 244
Körper 117, 139, 240

language of thought hypothesis *31*, 240–241, 248
Laplace, Pierre 161, 244
Leib (lived body) 117–118
localization 93, 241

male gaze 172, 241
Marr, David *28*, 222, 235
Maturana, Huberto *137*, 231, 238
mental representations chapter 3 *passim*, 67, 86, 88, *96*, 98–99, 100n7, 101, 103–104, 108, 111, 153, 166–168, 216, 241, 248
mentalese *31*, 241
Merleau-Ponty, Maurice 63n8, 209, 212, 235, 244
Mill, John Stuart 185, 240
Miller, George 28–29, 53, 86, 222, 233, 237
mindreading 213, 246–247
modality 85, 88–89, 97, 231, 242

neural reuse 92–96, 99, 105–106, 109–110, 143, 243
Neurath's Boat *83*, 181, 243
Noë, Alva *26*, *80*, 123, 152, 222

objective 187, 189, 198, 243
operant learning *23*, 232, 243
optic flow 124, 243

panpsychism 55, 64n16, 243
parity principle 55–56, 64n19, 68, **69**, 72–74, *75*, **81**, 83n2, 98, **151**, 201, 207–208, 233, 243
participatory sense-making 141n27, 192, 195, 218, 243
phenomenology 35, *134*, 141n25, 172, 209, 235, 237, 240, 244–245
physicalism *20*, 110n7, 242, 244–245
Plato xi, 9, 20, 39, *96*, 183, 199, 231, 246
poverty of the stimulus *23*, 243–244
psychology, autonomy of *20*, 231
Putnam, Hilary 24–25, 86, *109*, 234, 238
Pylyshyn, Zenon *28*, 249

Quine, Willard Van Orman *104*, 249

reliable coupling 53, 55–57, 59–60, 62, 64n18, 68, **69**, 72–74, 76, 81, 83n2, 114, **151**, 168, 200–204, 208–209, 211, 246
Ryle, Gilbert 36–37, 223, 226, 232, 238

scaffolding 53, 61, 210, 246
sense-making 118, 136–138, 141n27, 191–195, 197, 214, 218, 243, 246
Skinner, B.F. *23*, 164, 231–232, 243
space of possibilities 11, 16, 34, 58, 70, *81*, 83n1, 246
Strawson, Galen 166
Strawson, Peter 37–38, 223, 244
stress testing 68, **69**, **151**
symbol grounding problem 38–44, 46n10, 67, 102–104

tautology 17n1, 234, 247
theory of mind 46n12, 81, 147, 241, 246–247; *see also* mindreading
thick/thin concepts 61, *146*, 247
Thomas Reid *103*, 248
thought experiment 22, 36, 84n13, 91, 99, *109*, 161, 234, 238, 242, 248
transducer 87, 248
transeunt causation 159, 239, 248
Turing, Alan 22–24, 45n6, 46, 86, 97, 223, 230
Turing machine 24, 46n9
Turing Test 22, 24, 46, 248

Umwelt 118, 129–131, 138, 189, 193, 197, 240, 248

Varela, Francisco *137*, 147, 224, 231, 238
vehicles (of representation) 26–27, 88, 92, 234, 248
virtue 180–181, 183–185, 187–189, 191, 195, 197n4–197n5, 244, 246, 248

Wittgenstein, Ludwig 110n2, 139n2, 140n9, 238, 241
working memory 28–29, 53, 86, 237, 249

For Product Safety Concerns and Information please contact our EU representative GPSR@taylorandfrancis.com Taylor & Francis Verlag GmbH, Kaufingerstraße 24, 80331 München, Germany